Domestic Abuse Across the Lifespan: The Role of Occupational Therapy

Domestic Abuse Across the Lifespan: The Role of Occupational Therapy has been co-published simultaneously as *Occupational Therapy in Mental Health*, Volume 16, Numbers 3/4 2001.

Domestic Abuse Across the Lifespan: The Role of Occupational Therapy

Christine A. Helfrich, PhD, OTR/L
Editor

Domestic Abuse Across the Lifespan: The Role of Occupational Therapy has been co-published simultaneously as *Occupational Therapy in Mental Health*, Volume 16, Numbers 3/4 2001.

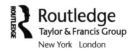
Routledge
Taylor & Francis Group
New York London

Domestic Abuse Across the Lifespan: The Role of Occupational Therapy has been co-published simultaneously as *Occupational Therapy in Mental Health*™, Volume 16, Numbers 3/4 2001.

First published by:

The Haworth Press, Inc., 10 Alice Street, Binghamton, NY 13904-1580 USA

This edition published 2012 by Routledge:

Routledge	Routledge
Taylor & Francis Group	Taylor & Francis Group
711 Third Avenue	2 Park Square, Milton Park
New York, NY 10017	Abingdon, Oxon OX14 4RN

Cover design by Thomas J. Mayshock Jr.

Library of Congress Cataloging-in-Publication Data

Domestic abuse across the lifespan : the role of occupational therapy / Christine A. Helfrich, editor.
    p. cm.
    "--co-published simultaneously as Occupational therapy in mental health, volume 16, numbers 3/4 2001".
    Includes bibliographical references and index.
    ISBN 0-7890-1384-3 (alk. paper)–ISBN 0-7890-1385-1 (alk. paper)
    1. Family violence–Prevention. 2. Occupational therapy. 3. Wife abuse–Prevention. I. Helfrich, Christine A.
RC569.5.F3 .D647 2001
616.85'822'06515–dc21   2001039148

Domestic Abuse Across the Lifespan: The Role of Occupational Therapy

CONTENTS

ABOUT THE EDITOR

Dr. Christine A. Helfrich, PhD, OTR/L, is currently Assistant Professor in the Department of Occupational Therapy at the University of Illinois at Chicago (UIC). Her scholarly interest is in psychosocial service provision, management, and consultation. She has taught in the areas of mental health, community practice, therapeutic use of self, culture and rehabilitation and disability in the urban environment.

Her current appointments include: Faculty Advisor in the Gender and Women's Studies Program at UIC; Editorial Board Member of the Occupational Therapy Journal of Research; member of the Faculty Advisory Committee for the Research Information Network on Women and Girls in Illinois; member of the Domestic Violence Coordinating Council of the Circuit Court of Cook County; Faculty Member, Collaborator and Advisory Board Member of the Mental Health Partnerships Project of the American Occupational Therapy Association; and Co-Chair of the Mental Health Special Interest Section of the Illinois Occupational Therapy Association.

Dr. Helfrich holds baccalaureate degrees in both Spanish and occupational therapy from Cleveland State University and a Master's of Science degree in occupational therapy from UIC. Her doctoral degree from UIC is in Public Health Community Health Science.

Dr. Helfrich has worked in mental health as both a clinician and as a consultant. Her interest in domestic violence as an issue for occupational therapy originated in her doctoral dissertation, and ethnographic study of homeless, abused women. She is currently the Principle Investigator on a field-initiated grant from the National Institute on Disability and Rehabilitation Research that seeks to explore the relationship between domestic violence and disability.

ABOUT THE CONTRIBUTORS

Ralph Adams, MS, OTR/L, is currently working in mental health practice at Portage Craigan Mental Health Center and is on the faculty at North Park College in Illinois. He has extensive experience in community mental health and academia.

Ann Aviles, OTR/L, received a Bachelor of Science in Occupational Therapy from the University of Illinois at Chicago, in 1998. She is currently a post-professional master's degree student in occupational therapy at UIC. She is working as a research assistant for Dr. Christine Helfrich. She is currently employed as a contingent staff therapist at Lutheran General Hospital working with the adult neurological rehabiliation population. She is also an adjunct faculty member at the University of Illinois at Chicago, Department of Occupational Therapy, teaching in the area of psychosocial occupational therapy intervention. Her interest in domestic violence centers on the family dynamics that result in adolescents becoming homeless and its effects on their ability to function.

Lara Collins, OTR/L, received a Bachelor of Science in Occupational Therapy from Wayne State University, College of Pharmacy and Allied Health, in 1993. She is currently a post-professional master's degree student in occupational therapy at the University of Illinois at Chicago. She is employed as a research assistant for Dr. Christine Helfrich at UIC. Prior to returning to graduate school, she was working full-time as a staff therapist in a pediatric outpatient setting. Her interest in domestic violence centers around its effects on children and family functioning.

Lisa Horita, OTR/L, received a Bachelor of Science in Occupational Therapy from the University of Illinois at Chicago, in 1998. She is currently working in adult rehabilitation. As a student, Lisa completed one of her fieldworks working with children who have witnessed domestic violence.

Jennifer L. Johnston, MS, OTR/L, received a Bachelor of Arts degree in Economics from DePauw University in Greencastle, Indiana and later earned a Master of Science in Occupational Therapy from Rush University in Chicago, Illinois. She is currently employed part-time as a pediatric occupational therapist at Therapeutic InterActions in LaGrange, Illinois, working with children with developmental delays due to problems such as sensory integrative disorder, cerebral palsy, autistic spectrum disorders, and Down Syndrome.

Mark Koch, OTR/L, received a Bachelor of Science in Occupational Therapy from the University of Missouri-Columbia in 1995. He is Program Director of the Coalition Against Rape and Domestic Violence (CARDV) in Fulton, Missouri, and a contract trainer for the Missouri Coalition Against Domestic Violence (MCADV). He has worked as an OT in forensic mental health, early childhood/school-based practice, and home health care. He is a member of the Network for Lesbian, Gay and Bisexual Concerns in Occupational Therapy and serves on the Board of Directors of the Missouri Victim Assistance Network (MoVA).

Shannon LaEace MacDonald, OTR/L, received a Bachelor of Science degree in Occupational Therapy at Xavier University in Cincinnati, Ohio. She is currently a graduate student at the University of Illinois at Chicago pursuing her master's degree in occupational therapy. She is employed at the Rehabilitation Institute of Chicago treating patients who have experienced neurological insults, burns, and cancer.

Mary Jean Lafata, OTR/L, received her Bachelor and Masters of Science degrees in Occupational Therapy from the University of Illinois at Chicago, with a minor in Women's Studies. Mary Jean has over a decade of experience in geriatrics and home health. Currently she is the director of a rehabilitation department in a long-term care facility for older adults. Her work with older adults raised her awareness of the prevalence of elder abuse, prompting her to focus her graduate studies on the development of the Occupational Therapy Elder Abuse Checklist.

Jonathan Nave, OTS, received a Bachelor of Arts with a double major in Biology and Chemistry and a minor in Global Studies from Drury College in Springfield, Missouri. He is currently a student at the University of Illinois at Chicago, seeking a master's degree in occupational therapy. Upon graduation, Jonathan intends to practice in pediatrics and early intervention in a community setting. He has a strong interest in seeing domestic violence end. He is also interested in the long-term effects of witnessing domestic violence and how occupational therapy intervention influences their outcomes.

Deborah Walens, MHPE, OTR/L, received her Masters in Health Professions Education from the University of Illinois at Chicago. She is currently Clinical Assistant Professor and Academic Fieldwork Coordinator at the University of Illinois at Chicago. She also works in two community agencies supervising level I and II fieldwork students in the areas of psychosocial rehabilitation and older adults. She is a Fellow of the American Occupational Therapy Association and chaired the AOTA-SIS Mental Health Education Task Force from 1992-94. Her interest in domestic abuse centers on the abuse of older adults and the education of occupational therapy students to work in settings that provide services to victims of abuse.

Introduction:
Domestic Abuse Across the Lifespan:
The Role of Occupational Therapy

This volume, *Domestic Abuse Across the Lifespan: The Role of Occupational Therapy*, was written to introduce a compilation of articles related to domestic violence. The profession of occupational therapy is poised to assume a position of leadership in working with victims of domestic abuse; however, many practitioners lack the skills and confidence needed to be effective with these emergent populations. This special publication provides a comprehensive overview of domestic abuse across the lifespan as well as theoretical and practical roles for occupational therapists.

The articles in this book cover a broad spectrum of domestic abuse including child abuse, intimate partner domestic violence and elder abuse. Most of the authors completed their work while graduate students in occupational therapy. All of the contributors provided feedback to each other during the development of this publication, which aided in consistency and comprehensiveness. Their articles overlap and the reader will find frequent references between individual articles. For educational purposes this document may be used in its entirety or each individual article may be used separately for specific populations. For that reason, the reader will notice occasional repetition of factual material between separate articles. Every attempt has been made to keep this repetition to a minimum.

Part I of this volume presents background knowledge necessary to

[Haworth co-indexing entry note]: "Introduction: Domestic Abuse Across the Lifespan: The Role of Occupational Therapy." Helfrich, Christine A. Co-published simultaneously in *Occupational Therapy in Mental Health* (The Haworth Press, Inc.) Vol. 16, No. 3/4, 2001, pp. 1-3; and: *Domestic Abuse Across the Lifespan: The Role of Occupational Therapy* (ed: Christine A. Helfrich) The Haworth Press, Inc., 2001, pp. 1-3. Single or multiple copies of this article are available for a fee from The Haworth Document Delivery Service [1-800-342-9678, 9:00 a.m. - 5:00 p.m. (EST). E-mail address: getinfo@haworthpressinc. com].

understand domestic abuse and the challenge of occupational therapists working with this population. The prevalence and demography of child abuse, partner violence and elder abuse are discussed in the first article. Discussion of the results of a research study, which surveyed occupational therapists to determine their knowledge and attitudes about domestic violence, follows.

Part II presents three articles discussing the role of occupational therapy working with victims of domestic violence. First, a framework for assessment and intervention is presented with case illustrations. Next, a student program developed to provide services to children who have been raised in abusive families is described. Finally, the role of occupational therapy as advocate for victims is illustrated through a case example provided by the director of a rape and domestic violence coalition.

Part III consists of three case applications illustrating the role of occupational therapy. The first article discusses and illustrates the role of occupational therapy on an inpatient rehabilitation unit with the child victim of Shaken Baby Syndrome and his family. Next, a case is presented illustrating the Occupational Therapy Psychosocial Assessment of Learning (OTPAL) with a child witness of domestic violence seen during a fieldwork rotation in a Before and After School Program for homeless abused families. Finally, the Occupational Therapy Elder Abuse Checklist is introduced with a case study demonstrating how the checklist was used to uncover elder abuse in a home health setting.

Together, this collection of articles provides the reader with a primer on domestic abuse across the lifespan. It is my hope that these articles will challenge therapists to examine their own beliefs and attitudes towards victims of abuse. The material and cases should raise readers' awareness of their attitudes and biases related to violence in our society. Through this awareness, therapists can change their practice to encompass the vast numbers of individuals who have been victimized. This victimization impacts their ability to function and to participate in desired, necessary and valued roles. These are certainly the concerns of occupational therapy. Occupational therapists must embrace these concerns and develop the skills needed to effectively empower individuals to engage in restoring function and involvement in life roles. It is only through empowerment that survivors of domestic abuse will develop the skills needed to live independently and to teach their children to communicate through non-violent means.

ACKNOWLEDGMENTS

This volume on domestic violence is a demonstration of the collaborative work of many individuals. I would like to especially acknowledge all of the women and children survivors of domestic violence who have shared their lives with my students and myself to help us understand the effects of violence in their lives. Next, I wish to thank the staff that works with victims of abuse for indulging all of us by allowing us to observe and question their work while we were learning ourselves.

While I have advised students on projects and theses related to domestic violence I did not envision a work such as this being published. Gary Kielhofner provided the encouragement to approach The Haworth Press about the idea of publishing a special collection on domestic violence. Mary Donohue and Marie-Louise Blount were open to this proposal and have provided much support and guidance as the publication came to fruition. Mary Donohue's availability and constant encouragement were invaluable. Each individual contributor provided collaborative feedback to each other and myself throughout the months prior to completion. Ann Aviles, Mary Jean Lafata, Shannon LaEace MacDonald and Deborah Walens participated in a writing group with me over several months to support the development of many of the articles in this collection. Ann Aviles, Meagan Cade, Lara Collins, Mrugaya Gorde and Carrie Schlosser worked endless hours editing, typing and formatting manuscripts to assist the authors. Their hard work, support, patience and humor made this document possible. Finally, the support and encouragement of my colleagues, friends and family encouraged me to bring this work and these ideas to publication for others to implement and critique. It is my hope that this document will encourage therapists to explore, question, critique and develop the role of occupational therapy with victims of domestic abuse.

Christine A. Helfrich, PhD, OTR/L

PART I

Domestic Abuse Across the Lifespan: Definitions, Identification and Risk Factors for Occupational Therapists

Christine A. Helfrich, PhD, OTR/L
Mary Jean Lafata, MS, OTR/L
Shannon LaEace MacDonald, OTR/L
Ann Aviles, OTR/L
Lara Collins, OTR/L

Christine A. Helfrich is Assistant Professor, Department of Occupational Therapy, University of Illinois at Chicago, 1919 W. Taylor Street (M/C 811), Chicago, IL 60612 (E-mail: *Helfrich@uic.edu*).

Mary Jean Lafata is an Occupational Therapist (E-mail: *mlafatal@aol.com*).

Shannon LaEace MacDonald is Staff Therapist, The Rehabilitation Institute of Chicago, 345 East Superior, Chicago, IL 60611 (E-mail: *SMACDONALD@rehabchicago. org*).

Ann Aviles is Research Assistant, Department of Occupational Therapy, University of Illinois at Chicago, Chicago, IL (E-mail: *aavile1@uic.edu*).

Lara Collins is Research Assistant, Department of Occupational Therapy, University of Illinois at Chicago, Chicago, IL (E-mail: *lcolli8@uic.edu*).

[Haworth co-indexing entry note]: "Domestic Abuse Across the Lifespan: Definitions, Identification and Risk Factors for Occupational Therapists." Helfrich, Christine A. et al. Co-published simultaneously in *Occupational Therapy in Mental Health* (The Haworth Press, Inc.) Vol. 16, No. 3/4, 2001, pp. 5-34; and: *Domestic Abuse Across the Lifespan: The Role of Occupational Therapy* (ed: Christine A. Helfrich) The Haworth Press, Inc., 2001, pp. 5-34. Single or multiple copies of this article are available for a fee from The Haworth Document Delivery Service [1-800-342-9678, 9:00 a.m. - 5:00 p.m. (EST). E-mail address: getinfo@haworthpressinc.com].

SUMMARY. Domestic abuse has reached epidemic proportions in the United States. Occupational therapists working in many different settings will encounter children, adults, elders and individuals with disabilities who have experienced intimate violence and abuse. This article presents common definitions and illustrative examples of each type of violence. Issues related to the difficulty inherent in identifying victims of abuse are discussed with an elaboration of indicators that are likely to be seen by an occupational therapist in the clinical setting. Risk factors for becoming a victim or an abuser for each population group and the effects of violence on victims are presented. A brief discussion of the legal and ethical implications of identifying and treating abuse victims concludes the article. *[Article copies available for a fee from The Haworth Document Delivery Service: 1-800-342-9678. E-mail address: <getinfo@haworthpressinc.com> Website: <http://www.HaworthPress.com> © 2001 by The Haworth Press, Inc. All rights reserved.]*

KEYWORDS. Domestic abuse, child abuse, domestic violence, elder abuse, occupational therapy and ethics

INTRODUCTION

Violence is a public health epidemic that impacts the field of occupational therapy. Of special concern within the larger problem of violence and injury are domestic violence against women and children, abuse of the elderly, and abuse and neglect of those with a disability. While no accurate estimate of the scale of domestic violence is available, imputations based on available evidence suggest a problem of considerable magnitude. For example, approximately half of all homicides involve individuals known to each other (Reiss & Roth, 1993) and abuse is the leading cause of death among infants and children (Peterson & Brown, 1994; Bethea, 1999). According to the National Crime Victimization Survey, approximately three-fourths of all violent events (e.g., rapes and assaults) involve an intimate or relative (U.S. Department of Justice, 1994). Injury is more likely to be sustained when assault involves an intimate, underscoring that domestic battery is a major vector for injury among women (Rosenberg & Mercy, 1991). Women, children, and the elderly appear to be at heightened risk for violent injury and a principal dynamic appears to be domestic abuse (U.S. Department of Justice, 1997). The Centers for Disease Control (CDC) estimated that 34% of American women are assaulted each year (CDC, 1993).

Up to four million women are abused each year with as many as two million suffering serious injury and 2,000-4,000 suffering death at the hands of their husbands, boyfriends, or former partners (Keller, 1996). Research indicates that domestic violence may be the leading cause of injury to women, resulting in more injuries that require medical intervention than rape, automobile accidents and muggings combined (Council on Ethical and Judicial Affairs, AMA, 1992).

Studies indicate that approximately 30% of all women who visit emergency rooms have injuries related to ongoing partner abuse (Abbott, Johnson, Koziol-McLain & Lowenstein, 1995; Dearwater, Coben, Campbell, Nah, McLoughlin & Bekemeier, 1998; Centers for Disease Control and Prevention, 1993). Of these battered women using emergency rooms, only 5% have been identified by staff as victims of domestic violence (Goldberg & Tomlanovich, 1984; Randall, 1990).

Child abuse has become a national concern. Reported cases of child abuse increased by 50% between 1985 and 1993 (Bethea, 1999). Abusing children has become an epidemic and has resulted in numerous children with disabilities. Astoundingly, each year 160,000 children suffer severe or life-threatening injury and 1,000-2,000 children die as a result of abuse (Bethea, 1999). Of those who die, 80% are under the age of five, and 40% are younger than one year of age (Starling, Holden & Jenny, 1995). Homicide is the fourth leading cause of death in children from one to four years of age and the third leading cause of death in children from five to fourteen (Bethea, 1999). It is widely accepted that a number of child abuse cases go underreported and that an accidental death may in fact have been a result of child abuse which was not closely investigated; therefore, the number of actual deaths from child abuse may be even higher.

Abuse of elders is also a concern. It has been estimated that 5% of the elderly population, or more than one million elders, are abused annually (U.S. Congress, 1990). Women are victims in a disproportionate amount of elder abuse cases. Seventy-five percent of the incidents of psychological abuse and 92% of financial abuse/exploitation cases of elder abuse that are reported are abuse of female elders (Butler, 1999). The oldest elders in our population (age 80 and over) are abused and neglected at two to three times their proportion of the elderly population (National Center on Elder Abuse, 1998). This abuse often goes unreported, with estimates that only one in eight cases is reported to authorities (Larue, 1992; U.S. Congress, 1990).

The National Elder Abuse Incidence Study (NEAIS) report suggests that at least one-half million older persons in domestic settings (those housed in institutions were not included in this study) were abused and/or neglected, or experienced self-neglect during 1996 (National Center on Elder Abuse, 1998). For every reported incident of elder abuse, neglect, or self-neglect, approximately five go unreported (National Center on Elder Abuse, 1998).

Estimates of the incidence of abuse and neglect during 1996 from the NEAIS are lower than other previous estimates. The report indicates that it is difficult to directly compare results across various studies because of significant differences in research objectives, designs and methodologies. Some studies examined the prevalence of elder abuse (i.e., the total number of cases of abuse in a given population at a designated time), while others studied the incidence (i.e., the number of new cases of abuse occurring over a specific time period). Prevalence studies provide larger estimates. Definitions of abuse and neglect, research time frames and geographic areas vary considerably across studies, making direct comparison impossible (National Center on Elder Abuse, 1998).

Reports of abuse of the elderly population first appeared in writing about 25 years ago. Researchers quickly began to attempt to determine the prevalence and scope of the problem. The biggest problem in the research of elder abuse is the lack of a widely accepted definition of abuse. The lack of a definition of abuse not only can cause professionals to miss potential abusive situations but also may perpetuate the poor funding levels associated with this problem. According to a report by the U.S. Congress (1990), states spend only $3.80 per resident for protective services for elders as opposed to the $45 per resident for child protective services (U.S. Congress, 1990).

Abuse of people with disabilities is another national concern. Due to their increased dependence on others, women with disabilities are even more vulnerable to domestic violence than women without disabilities. Women with disabilities in both Canada and the United States identify violence as their number one concern (Rivers-Moore, 1999; Berkley Planning Associates, 1996). These women are often dependent on their abuser for affection, communication, financial support, physical support and/or medical support (Rivers-Moore, 1999). Therefore, reporting the abuse may result in more severe negative consequences. Women may risk loss of accessible housing, poverty, further institutionalization and the loss of their children. Because of their disability, these women may not have access to literature that describes support services that are available, or may not have access to transportation to the building or access into the building where services are housed (Rivers-Moore, 1999).

The findings are inconsistent in the literature regarding the incidence of abuse of women with disabilities compared to those without disabilities. In a study of 946 women (504–disabled, 442–non-disabled) conducted by The Center for Research on Women with Disabilities (CROWD), 62% of both groups reported incidences of abuse. There also was no difference in the incidence of both groups when abuse was broken down into emotional, physical and sexual abuse. A husband was the perpetrator in 26% of both groups (Nosek & Howland, 1998). In contrast to that study, other sources indicate that women with disabilities regardless of age, race, ethnicity, sexual orientation, or class are assaulted, raped, and abused at a rate twice that of women without disabilities (U.S. Department of Justice, 1997-98). The CROWD study found significant differences in the duration of abuse before the woman left her partner. Women with disabilities endured abuse for 3.9 years on average compared to 2.5 years for women without disabilities (Nosek & Howland, 1998). It is well documented that abuse increases in severity and lethality over time (Walker, 1994), thus placing women with disabilities at greater risk for severe injury or death.

DEFINING DOMESTIC VIOLENCE

Practitioners who lack a clear understanding of domestic violence may under-identify or fail to report such information. Legal definitions of domestic violence vary from state to state; however, most definitions incorporate similar information. Readers should consult their state's Domestic Violence Act for a complete definition. For the purposes of this article the following definition will be used:

> Domestic violence is any act carried out with the intention of physically or emotionally harming another person who is related to you by blood, present or prior marriage, or common law marriage, having (or having had) a child in common, or having (or

having had) a dating relationship. This also includes a person with a disability and their personal assistant. Domestic violence includes physical abuse, sexual abuse, emotional abuse, economic abuse, destruction of property or pets and stalking. (Illinois Domestic Violence Act of 1986)

This definition includes partner abuse, elder abuse, child abuse and abuse of individuals with a disability by a family member or by their personal assistant who may not be a relative. In this article each type of abuse will be addressed separately. Unless otherwise indicated, this article will consider the domestic violence victim to be an adult female and the perpetrator to be an adult male. Child abuse or maltreatment includes "physical abuse, sexual abuse, psychological abuse, and general, medical, and educational neglect" (Bethea, 1999). Elder abuse is defined by state laws. State definitions vary as to what constitutes the abuse, neglect, or exploitation of the elderly; however, the definition for abuse/neglect of the elderly is divided into three categories: domestic, institutional and self-neglect/self-abuse.

As described in the definition there are six types of domestic abuse. For clarity, they will first be discussed in general terms, followed by specific definitions for the elderly and those individuals with disabilities.

- *Physical Abuse.* Someone who is being or has been physically abused may have endured any of the following: hitting, punching, kicking, biting, being thrown or tied down, choking, smothering, burning, being threatened with a weapon, refusal of help when sick or injured, and/or being driven recklessly to frighten her. She may have also been victim to the unwarranted administration of drugs, physical restraints, force feeding, and/or physical punishment of any kind.
- *Emotional Abuse.* Someone who is being or has been emotionally abused may have endured any of the following: verbal abuse, intimidation, threats, isolation, restriction of activities, humiliation, insults, ignoring of needs, lying, and/or breaking promises.
- *Sexual Abuse.* Someone who is being or has been sexually abused may have endured any of the following: being forced to have sex, injury during sex, weapons used intravaginally, orally or anally, coerced to have sex without protection, sexual criti-

cism, or flaunting extra-marital affairs. Sexual contact with any person unable to consent is also considered sexual abuse.

- *Economic Abuse.* Someone who is being economically abused may have endured any of the following: having money taken away, being prevented from getting or keeping a job, and/or being made to ask for money. Economic abuse also includes misused or misappropriated money or assets that result in a disadvantage to the victim and/or the profit of someone else. Examples include, being forced to turn over money or property, a signature being forged, misused or stolen money or possessions, being coerced or deceived into signing a document, and the improper use of guardianship, conservatorship, or power of attorney.
- *Destruction of Property or Pets.* This includes the breaking of property or her favorite objects, hurting or killing her pets or giving away objects.
- *Stalking.* Someone who is being stalked is being followed, placed under surveillance, or the subject of any conduct which places her in reasonable apprehension of immediate or future bodily harm, sexual assault, confinement or restraint.

The following additional definitions are appropriate when a person is reliant on a caregiver, either as an elder or secondary to a disability. When this refers to both elders and a person with a disability, dependent is used for ease of reading and to signify reliance on assistance. However, it does not imply complete dependence.

- *Physical Abuse.* In addition to the general definition, a dependent is considered to be physically abused if they are assaulted, are moved with rough or inappropriate handling, receive inappropriate personal or medical care, experience over-use of restraint, are a subject of inappropriate behavior modification, are over-medicated, and/or confined.
- *Neglect.* A person is considered neglected if the caregiver fails to provide the elder with life's necessities. The neglect may be intentional, when a caregiver deliberately fails his/her responsibilities in order to punish the elder. Examples include willfully withholding medicines, food, or water. The neglect may also be unintentional resulting from ignorance or a genuine inability to complete the task. Examples include not changing a dependent's incontinence supplies frequently enough, resulting in decubitus

ulcers, or being forcibly confined or restrained. Self-neglect is defined as a dependent withholding food, medicine, medical treatment or personal care necessary for well-being. Examples include not taking prescribed medications or refusing medical treatment.

- *Abandonment.* The desertion of a dependent by an individual who has assumed responsibility for providing care, or physical custody.
- *Violation of Rights.* A person's rights are considered violated when she is: being forced out of one's home or being forced into another setting without due process; being deprived of the right to move freely, without physical restraints; being deprived of adequate and appropriate medical treatment; having one's property taken without due process of law; being deprived of a clean and safe environment; having the right to privacy denied; or being deprived of freedom from verbal abuse. The right to complain or have grievances addressed is also an inalienable right (U.S. Congress, 1990). In addition to these rights, according to Quinn and Tomita (1986), violation of rights also includes being denied the right or opportunity to vote, attend church, or open one's own personal mail. Denial or violation of these rights is a form of abuse, which is reportable. Many of the rights listed above were included in other definitions of abuse mentioned above.
- *Emotional.* In addition to the general definition of emotional abuse, a dependent is considered to be a victim of emotional abuse when she is being treated like an infant. Emotional deprivation, denial of the right to make personal decisions, and threats of having one's children taken away are also considered emotional abuse.
- *Sexual Abuse.* In addition to the general definition, a dependent is considered to be a victim of sexual abuse when touching, fondling or any other sexual activity occurs when the person is unable to understand, unwilling to consent, threatened or physically forced. A woman with a disability is considered to be a victim of sexual abuse if others deny her sexuality, deny her the opportunity to receive sexual information/education (e.g., about birth control and childbirth), is a subject of verbal harassment regarding

sex. Forced abortion or sterilization is also considered sexual abuse.

• *Isolation.* A person is considered to be isolated when she is excluded or kept away from family, friends or regular activities. Giving a dependent the "silent treatment" and enforced social isolation are also examples of emotional and/or psychological abuse.

The types of abuse described indicate a continuum of behaviors and actions that may not always be indicative of abuse. In every relationship there are disagreements and quarrels. Who defines abuse? The general rule is to allow the *woman* to define whether or not an act is abusive. The health care practitioner's role is to educate the woman regarding the legal definition of abuse and inform her of legal and practical options (Sassetti, 1993). She must then make a decision of what she will do based on the information she has been given. The victim of abuse has to experience only one type of abuse to be identified as a victim and protected under her state's domestic violence act. Lafata and Helfrich (2001) provide a thorough discussion of the added challenges of defining neglect of those persons who are dependent.

Later in this article specific legal and ethical implications for the occupational therapist working with victims of abuse will be discussed.

IDENTIFICATION OF ABUSE VICTIMS

There are a number of reasons why battered women have gone unidentified. Studies have divided the reasons into three general areas: (a) health care providers' reluctance to screen for domestic violence, (b) women's reluctance to disclose domestic violence and (c) lack of staff training for how to screen for domestic violence.

Reluctance to Screen for Domestic Violence

Health care providers have offered a wide range of impediments to identification of abuse. There has been a tradition within the health care system of interpreting domestic violence as a private matter, or a "taboo topic" (Hoff, 1992; Keller, 1996). Many professionals also hold the belief that battered women may be masochistic, and fall into a pattern of "blaming the victim" (Gremillion & Kanof, 1996; Holtz & Furniss, 1993; Keller, 1996).

Providers may also label victims as "difficult patients" when they appear to be passive, hostile, anxious, depressed, hysterical, or engaging in substance abuse (Holtz & Furniss, 1993; Kurz, 1987). Providers are more likely to respond to a battered woman when they see the woman as a "true victim," for example, a woman with a pleasant personality who claims to be taking action to leave the violent relationship (Kurz, 1987). Health care professionals also report that the identification and referral of battered women involves too much of their time, and because they may underestimate the prevalence of abuse, they may not look at it as a worthwhile investment of time (Gremillion & Kanof, 1996). Becoming involved with an abused patient may have a psychological impact on the providers, especially if they have been involved in partner or spousal abuse themselves (Gremillion & Kanof, 1996; Quillian, 1996). Other reasons why health care professionals fail in identification may be a concern over offending the patient, a feeling of powerlessness to respond, a fear of being involved with the law, concern over misidentification, and a reluctance to see domestic violence as a medical issue (Ferris, 1994; Neufield, 1996).

Women's Reluctance to Disclose Domestic Violence

Women also may fail to spontaneously self-disclose a history of abuse for numerous underlying psychological, social, and institutional reasons. Abused women may fear bodily harm or death from the perpetrator if they disclose the abuse. Many abused women also present with psychological vulnerability and low self-esteem and may be embarrassed or ashamed of the abusive situation (Rodriguez, Quiroga & Bauer, 1996). Abused women may feel a sense of family responsibility, fulfilling the traditional gender role of protecting the spouse and fearing intervention in the family by the authorities. The perceived and real difficulties of single parenthood and economic insecurity may also be reasons why abused women do not identify themselves. Many battered women may not self-identify themselves as abused because they do not understand the definition of domestic violence (Keller, 1996; Rodriguez et al., 1996).

Staff Untrained to Screen for Domestic Violence

A significant reason why many professionals do not appropriately identify these women is a lack of knowledge and training regarding domestic violence (Neufield, 1996). Training in domestic violence and in how to make routine inquiries to determine probable domestic violence is still rare in health care settings, even those that tend to see high proportions of women experiencing abuse (Keller, 1996).

Although most existing domestic violence data are derived from emergency department studies, these studies may not present a representative sample of the general population of battered women (Sugg & Inui, 1992). Victims of domestic violence also seek services in primary care clinics and physician's offices. Battered women account for 14-28% of women attending primary care clinics (Gin, Rucker, Frayne, Cypan & Hubbell, 1991; Rath, Jarratt & Leonardson, 1989). Women who are abused visit their primary care physician more often than women who are not abused (Elliott & Johnson, 1995). Cases seen in these settings most often do not involve recent physical trauma but rather present with stress-related illnesses and complaints such as chronic pain, sleep disturbances, frequent headaches, and abdominal and gynecologic problems (Koss, 1993). It is of note that most research in medical settings has taken place in urban emergency departments where poor, minority populations are likely to go for primary care which may inflate the prevalence of domestic violence for minority groups (Holtz & Furniss, 1993).

Occupational Therapists' Identification of Abuse

Occupational therapists are also reluctant to identify or work with victims of domestic violence. Consistent with the literature on other health care providers, Johnston, Adams, and Helfrich (2001) found that occupational therapists' knowledge about domestic abuse correlated directly with their attitudes about occupational therapy's role with victims. In a study of over 200 practicing occupational therapists Johnston et al. (2001) found that therapists were able to correctly answer only 65% of basic knowledge questions related to the identification and treatment of domestic violence victims. Sixty-eight percent of therapist respondents stated they did not feel adequately prepared to identify victims of domestic abuse. However, 88% indicated that they have a low acceptance of violence towards women, which is a finding consistent with occupational therapy's code of ethics. The individual therapist's level of knowledge about wife abuse was directly correlated to the degree of caring attitude they expressed about victims of abuse and to their views about the role that occupational therapy should have with victims of abuse. Other factors that contributed to more knowledge of abuse or a more positive attitude towards working with abuse victims included being female, being abused as a child, and receiving formal instruction regarding domestic abuse. These factors are consistent with studies of attitudes of other health care professionals. The level of education received by occupational therapists regarding wife abuse was very low. Only 35% reported having received any formal instruction on this topic. Each reader of this article will be contributing to a change in the field of occupational therapy where more practitioners are informed about domestic violence.

Occupational therapists have ample opportunity to discover suspected mistreatment or abuse of elders. However, a search of the archives of the *American Journal of Occupational Therapy* uncovered only one article dealing with the abuse of the elderly. This article was entitled *Ethical Dilemmas in Family Caregiving for the Elderly: Implications for Occupational Therapy*. This article did not directly deal with abuse of the elderly but with ethical issues related to caring for an elder. These issues revolved around exploring the client's ethical beliefs to assist in maximizing the therapeutic relationship (Hasselkus, 1991). In general, professionals fail to detect abuse and lack awareness of the high risk factors of abuse (Kosberg, 1988). Lack of awareness is complicated by an often subtle presentation of the abuse (e.g., poor hygiene and dehydration), disbelief that abuse is taking place, fear of jeopardizing a relationship with a caregiver and requests by the elder that the doctor not report the abuse (patient/physician privilege) (Swagerty, Takahashi & Evans, 1999).

When occupational therapists work with children who are victims of abuse and/or neglect they may not be prepared to identify or understand behaviors they exhibit. Children may withdraw socially, demonstrate oppositional or aggressive behavior, lie and/or steal (American Medical Association, 2000). Occupational therapists, who most likely are seeing the child for reasons other than abuse, are not necessarily prepared to work with these children effectively.

Occupational therapists receive little preparation for dealing with the effects of violence. The Mental Health Special Interest Section

(MHSIS): Education Task Force Report (Walens, Dickie, Tomlinson, Raynor, Wittman & Kannenberg, 1995) found that few fieldwork facilities are willing to incorporate psychosocial goals into traditional rehabilitative programs. Therefore, if a client is initially referred for a physical impairment, but also has psychosocial issues, very few students have the opportunity or encouragement to pursue these issues as goals. This limits the occupational therapist's ability to treat the whole patient. Respondents to the MHSIS study also found that students often lacked preparation for "real world" types of psychosocial issues that an occupational therapist might encounter (Walens et al., 1995). There are concerns that students do not know how to deal with issues of sexual abuse, the potential violence of clients, the need for self-defense and community based programming (Walens et al., 1995). In general, the study found that occupational therapists are not equipped to deal with psychosocial issues that may override the client's physical needs.

THE VICTIMS OF DOMESTIC VIOLENCE

Contrary to many myths and stereotypes, domestic violence is not partial to demographics, age, socioeconomic status, race or ethnicity. The only risk factor for becoming an adult victim of domestic violence is being female (Sassetti, 1993). In 95% of domestic violence cases the woman is the victim. However, there are several events that occur in a woman's life that place her at higher risk for becoming a victim of abuse (American Medical Association, 1992). These include:

- History of being abused as a child
- Beginning cohabitation with a partner
- Legally marrying
- Pregnancy (increases the risk by 25%)
- Separation from military service (self or partner)
- Loss of a job (self or partner)
- New signs of independence by the woman (i.e., new job, return to school, graduation from school)
- Separation or divorce

Each of these life events threatens the status quo of the current relationship. This may require a renegotiation of roles between partners, which is the dynamic believed to increase the risk for abuse. In most abusive relationships the partner has a strong need to be in control. His control is in jeopardy during times of change in the relationship. The woman's risk of being abused does not end when she leaves the relationship. In fact, she is at most risk for being killed after she has left her abusive partner (Russell, 1995). The Chicago Women's Health Risk Study (CWHRS, 2000) recorded the violent events that occurred in 497 women's lives in the previous year. The results showed that a total of 85% of the women who had experienced severe violence had also left or attempted to end the relationship. Sixty-six percent of women who had experienced less severe incidents of violence had left or attempted to end the relationship (CWHRS, 2000). The CWHRS (2000) also found that for 40% of women homicide victims in this study, an immediate precipitating factor of the fatal incident was the woman leaving or trying to end the relationship.

In addition to the direct victims of domestic violence (the actual target or recipient of abuse), there are also indirect victims. Indirect victims are those individuals who have witnessed the abuse of another family member or whose lives are directly impacted by the abuse of a family member. This includes children who were present while their mother was being abused. The children may experience psychological (e.g., depression) or behavioral (e.g., aggression) effects or they may be affected by the decisions that are made as a result of the abuse (e.g., loss of custody). In order to escape the abusive relationship the family may need to go into a shelter or move away. The child is forced to change schools, meet new friends, lose or change their contact with the other parent, and adapt to a new environment and lifestyle. While this is occurring the child is trying to integrate a myriad of feelings and experiences with a mother who is doing the same to adjust to the effects of the violence.

When children become direct victims, the abuse is labeled child abuse and there are a number of factors that increase a child's risk of becoming a victim. A child who is born to a parent who is inadequately prepared for parenting, a teenager, a substance abuser, has poor coping skills or is under stress, is more likely to be abused (Duhaime, Christian, Rorke & Zummerman, 1998; Lacey, 1998). If the child is one of a multiple birth (i.e., twins) or whose family has multiple children under the age of 18 months, they are at greater risk for abuse (Duhaime et al., 1998; Lacey, 1998). Characteristics of an infant also put them at greater risk. Children who are difficult to soothe or calm, children born prematurely or of a low birth weight and children who have disabilities are at a greater risk of becoming abused (Bethea, 1999; Duhaime et al., 1998; Lacey, 1998). Older children who exhibit difficulties with social interaction and overall general functioning also are at greater risk for abuse (Belsky & Vondra, 1989). Economic issues also play a role. If the child is born to a family that lives in economic strains or poverty, they are more likely to be abused than those who do not live in those circumstances (Duhaime et al., 1998; Lacey, 1998). All of the factors that can increase a child's risk of becoming a victim of abuse can occur either in isolation or with a combination of other factors.

THE EFFECTS OF DOMESTIC VIOLENCE

The domestic violence literature suggests twelve indicators that aid in identifying abuse. They are: (1) Depressive symptoms; (2) Suicidal ideation or attempts; (3) Anxiety symptoms; (4) Chronic pain in back, pelvic region (obstetrical or gynecological manifestations), chest, or neck; (5) Unexplained traumatic injury; (6) Fractures in various stages of healing; (7) Somatic disorders, such as sleep disturbance, appetite disturbance, and gastrointestinal problems; (8) Alcohol or drug abuse; (9) Chronic use of pain medication or sleeping pills; (10) Child abuse, by either parent; (11) Alcohol abuse or depression or antisocial personality disorder in husband; and (12) History of abuse in either partner (Gerlock, 1999; Keller, 1996).

Domestic violence has both short and long-term effects on the individual. Short-term effects of domestic violence may include emotional or physical injury or disability, interference with role function, economic difficulty and homelessness. Long-term effects may include continued physical or mental disability, loss of role identity, loss of family ties and support systems, loss of employment, homelessness and in the most severe cases, death may ultimately occur. Most studies looking at the medical effects of domestic violence only address the immediate, acute effects; studies that explore the long-term consequences related to disability are needed.

Many women who experience domestic violence have children who are also living in an abusive household. Domestic violence in the home not only affects the woman being battered, it also has an impact on the children living in these situations. Children in this situation may be exposed to threats of violence, may overhear the violence, and/or they may visually witness the violence. It has been estimated that at least 3.3 million children witness physical and verbal spousal abuse each year (Osofsky, 1995). It has also been noted that in homes where domestic violence occurs, children are physically abused and neglected at a rate 15 times higher than the national average. The unpredictable home environment is extremely stressful to normal child development. This has implications on their social, psychological, educational and physical development (Thormaehlen & Bass-Feld, 1994).

Children who have been exposed to violence show a variety of symptoms, beginning as early as infancy (Nelms, 1994). Children who are exposed to violence exhibit feelings of guilt, shame, lack of trust, poor self-esteem, helplessness and hopelessness (Thormaehlen & Bass-Feld, 1994). Children's ability to cope and the behaviors they exhibit may differ depending upon their age. Numerous studies have documented that although very young children may not understand the violence, they are likely to exhibit emotional distress, immature behavior, somatic complaints, and regressions in toileting and language (Osofsky, 1995).

School-aged children may better understand acts of violence and the intentions behind them. Children at this age may exhibit post-traumatic stress disorder, exhibit a greater frequency of externalizing aggressive/delinquent behavior or may become withdrawn/anxious (Osofsky, 1995). The child's overall functioning, social competency, and school performance may also be affected negatively.

Adolescents who have been exposed to violence (especially over a long period of time) demonstrate high levels of aggression, acting out, anxiety, behavior problems, school problems, truancy, feelings of hopelessness and revenge seeking (Osofsky, 1995). Children at this stage in life may also attach themselves to peer groups and gangs as a substitute family. Witnessing domestic violence not only affects a child's development, it also teaches children that violence is a problem-solving method.

Children exposed to violence may rely on violence as a method of dealing with disputes or frustration (Osofsky, 1995). This has implications on their ability to cope in stressful situations, and during social interactions. Children who have been exposed to violence may turn inward, becoming emotionally withdrawn or disconnected, resulting in an inability to discuss their feelings with others. Children may come to view violence as an acceptable way to resolve conflicts. This will have long-term effects on their ability to form relationships and exhibit healthy coping abilities. Witnessing domestic violence teaches children that violence is a part of family relationships, perpetrators of violence in intimate relationships often go unpunished, and that violence is a means to control other people (Massachusetts Coalition of Battered Women's Service Group and The Children's Working Group, 1995).

Child Abuse

The disabling conditions following child abuse are vast. Children not only suffer acutely from the physical and mental cruelty of child abuse; they experience many long-term deficits. Bethea (1999) reported that children who are abused experience delays in reaching developmental milestones, chronic neurologic disabilities, refusal to attend school and separation anxiety disorders. Being a victim of child abuse can also increase the likelihood of future substance abuse, aggressive behaviors, high-risk health behaviors, criminal activity, somatization, depressive and affective disorders, personality disorders, post-traumatic stress disorder, panic attacks and schizophrenia (Bethea, 1999; Britton, 1998). Adults who have experienced abuse as a child are more likely to abuse their own children or spouse (Bethea, 1999; Olds, Henderson, Kitzman & Cole, 1995).

Elder Abuse

Elder abuse has several emotional and behavioral consequences and is associated with shorter survival rates. The elder may become withdrawn or passive or may demonstrate increased overall fear (Lafata & Helfrich, 2001). In a study designed to evaluate the mortality of elders whose abuse had been reported and corroborated, elder mistreatment and self-neglect were associated with shorter survival rates, after controlling for other factors that increase mortality in elders (Lachs, Williams, O'Brien, Pillemar & Charlston, 1998) (See Table 1).

INDICATORS OF DOMESTIC ABUSE

In most cases the women, children or dependents seen in occupational therapy that are victims of domestic abuse will be referred for reasons other than abuse. Therefore, it is important, not only to know what questions to ask to screen for victimization, but also, to know what visible signs to look for. The following is a table that provides examples of signs that may indicate abuse (see Table 2).

Occupational therapists are often in a position to see these physical indicators because of the nature of their relationships with clients. Occupational therapists evaluate a person's observed ability to perform, rather than basing their evaluation solely on the person's report of their performance. Therefore, in the course of evaluating a woman's ability to complete Activities of Daily Living, she is more likely to visibly expose injuries, which would not be visible to a social worker asking about her discharge plans. The occupational therapist, upon seeing an unusual injury, is challenged by what to do with that information. It is common to dismiss an injury or bruise as insignificant or not out of the ordinary. Many of the injuries listed above could also occur through accidents. So, how does the occupational therapist decide if the injury warrants further exploration? The following questions may help to clarify the therapist's level of concern about the possibility that an injury is abuse-related.

1. Is the type of injury consistent with the explanation of the cause? (Black eyes don't usually occur from running into a wall)
2. Is there a central pattern to the injuries? (Torso, breasts)
3. Are there bruises in various stages of healing? (Bruises change color over a period of time)
4. Is the woman trying to keep the injury hidden? (Wearing long sleeves in the summer to cover up lacerations on her arm)
5. Does the individual become dismissive or defensive when questioned about the injury? ("It's nothing," or "It was just an accident!")
6. Is the injury consistent with the individual's developmental level?

Lafata and Helfrich (2001) discuss the process for assessing for elder abuse in detail. They provide a checklist with guidelines for use by the occupational therapist.

An occupational therapist may also have the opportunity to identify

TABLE 1. Elder Abuse Risk Factors

RISK TYPE	FACTORS THAT INCREASE RISK OF ABUSE
Intrapersonal risks (Ferguson & Beck, 1983; Henton et al., 1984; Larue, 1992; Pillemer & Finkelhor, 1988; U.S. Congress, 1990; Lachs & Pillemer, 1995)	■ Physical and/or mental disability, dependence on others and poor health ■ Female sex ■ Aged older than 75 ■ Depression, feelings of hopelessness and uselessness ■ Living with others ■ Drinking problem
Interpersonal (Larue, 1992; U.S. Congress, 1990; Kosberg, 1988)	■ Lack of family support ■ Substance abuse problems ■ Excessive dependence on the elder for financial assistance, housing or other necessities ■ History of violence or antisocial behavior ■ Unresolved parent-child conflict ■ Inexperience as a caregiver ■ Marital conflict ■ Need to retaliate for past grievances, real or imagined
Situational (Ferguson & Beck, 1983; Kosberg, 1981)	■ Overcrowding of the home ■ Caregiver isolation from peers or family ■ Lack of respite for primary caregiver ■ Financial strain ■ Inclusion of the elder into a family with existing difficulties present
Sociocultural	■ Ageism (negative feelings toward the aging) ■ Small family size (limiting the ability to share responsibility for care)

child abuse. It is not only important to look for the physical signs of abuse (stated previously), it is also important to look for atypical behaviors that may suggest the presence of physical, sexual, and/or substance abuse (Kurtz et al., 1996). Some of these atypical behaviors and psychosocial issues that children who are experiencing abuse may demonstrate are: depression, low self-esteem, loss of trust, anxiety, denial, problems with intimacy, feelings of having no future, and distortion of the family (Kurtz, Hick-Coolick, Jarvis & Kurtz, 1996).

TABLE 2. Indicators of Abuse

Type of Abuse	Indicator of Abuse
Physical Abuse (King & Ryan, 1989; Moss & Taylor, 1991; National Center on Elder Abuse, 1998)	■ Bruises in unusual places (back of arm, breast or genitals), bruises at various stages of healing (indicating repetitive pattern of injury), welts, black eyes, untreated injuries, open wounds, punctures. ■ Burns caused by cigarettes, ropes, "dry burns" caused by irons or stoves, particularly in unusual places (the back) or of prolonged severity. ■ Lacerations to the facial area (lips, eyes) or genitals. ■ Orthopedic injuries that do not fit the individual's developmental level or explanation (spiral fracture to the arm explained by falling down stairs), strains and/or dislocations. ■ Head & facial injuries such as subdural hematomas (caused by shaking or hitting), absence of hair, retinal and jaw injuries, skull fractures. ■ Internal injuries including injury to an unborn fetus caused by external trauma to the stomach area. ■ Broken eyeglasses/frames, physical signs of being subjected to punishment or signs of being restrained. ■ Laboratory findings of medical overdose or underutilization of prescribed medications. ■ Reports of being slapped or mistreated. ■ Sudden change of behavior. ■ Refusal of the caregiver to allow visitors to see the dependent alone.
Sexual Abuse (National Center on Elder Abuse, 1998)	■ Bruises around the breast or genital area. ■ Unexplained venereal disease or genital infections. ■ Unexplained vaginal or anal bleeding. ■ Torn, stained or bloody underclothing. ■ Being sexually assaulted or raped.
Emotional/Psychological Abuse (National Center on Elder Abuse, 1998)	■ Emotional upset or agitation. ■ Extreme withdrawal and non-communicative or non-responsiveness. ■ Being verbally or emotionally mistreated.
Neglect (National Center on Elder Abuse, 1998)	■ Dehydration, malnutrition, untreated bedsores and/or poor personal hygiene. ■ Unattended or untreated health problems. ■ Hazardous or unsafe living conditions. ■ Unsanitary or unclean living conditions. ■ A dependent's report of being neglected.

TABLE 2 (continued)

Type of Abuse	Indicator of Abuse
Self-neglect (National Center on Elder Abuse, 1998)	■ Dehydration, malnutrition, untreated or improperly attended medical conditions, and poor personal hygiene. ■ Hazardous or unsafe living conditions. ■ Unsanitary or unclean living conditions. ■ Inappropriate and/or inadequate clothing, lack of necessary medical aids. ■ Grossly inadequate housing or homelessness.
Abandonment (National Center on Elder Abuse, 1998)	■ The desertion of a dependent at a hospital, nursing facility or other similar institution. ■ The desertion of a dependent at a shopping mall or other public location. ■ A dependent's own report of being abandoned.
Financial or Material Exploitation (National Center on Elder Abuse, 1998)	■ Sudden changes in a bank account or banking practice, including an unexplained withdrawal of large sums of money by a person accompanying the elder. ■ The inclusion of additional names on an elder's bank signature card. ■ Unauthorized withdrawal of funds using an elder's ATM card. ■ Abrupt changes in a will or other financial documents. ■ Unexplained disappearance of funds or valuable possessions. ■ Provisions of substandard care or bills unpaid despite the availability of adequate funds. ■ The provision of services that are not necessary. ■ Discovery of an elder's signature forged for financial transactions or for the titles of the elder's possessions. ■ Sudden appearance of previously uninvolved relatives claiming rights to an elder's affairs and possessions. ■ Unexplained sudden transfer of assets to a family member or someone outside of the family. ■ An elder's report of financial exploitation.

It is difficult to identify psychological and behavioral indicators of abuse. Part of the difficulty arises from the fact that the indicators are often the same as the effects of domestic abuse on one's psychosocial functioning described earlier such as guilt, self-doubt, denial, fear, dissociation, anger, shame and helplessness (Stark & Flitcraft, 1996). These indicators may also be present in women who have suffered other types of psychological trauma. In order to avoid errant labeling of women, the occupational therapist is encouraged to ask questions directly leading to understanding if abuse has played a role in the current presentation.

RISK FACTORS FOR BECOMING AN ABUSER

The risk factors for becoming an abuser are speculatory. Occupational therapists are likely to be in situations of identifying individuals (parents and caregivers) who are at risk for becoming perpetrators of child and elder abuse. Those at risk for child abuse are likely to be identified by therapists working with children and also by therapists working with adults who are under extreme stress and have children or parents at home to care for. In addition, therapists working in home health may have the opportunity to assess risk of elder abuse by the individual's partner, grown children, or caregiver. Treatment of partners who abuse is very risky and involvement with the abuser directly may place the women at greater risk for violence.

There is no consensus as to the psychological makeup of an abusive partner; however, results from Gondolf's (1988) study using the Millon Clinical Multiaxial Inventory-III revealed that 25% exhibited severe mental disorders, 25% exhibited narcissistic personality traits, 24% exhibited passive aggressive traits and 19% were clinically depressed. This study also demonstrated that over half of the men had abused alcohol (Gondolf, 1988). Healy, Smith and O'Sullivan (1998) identify three different types of batterers. The "Family Only" batterer is one who is described as a perfectionist, conforming and with little social skills. The "Dysphoric/Borderline" batterer is emotional, experienced parental rejection and fears abandonment. And, the "Generally Violent/Antisocial" batterer tends to abuse alcohol, lacks empathy, has rigid gender role attitudes and is narcissistic (Healy et al., 1998).

Child Abuse

Early findings suggested that women were often the perpetrators of fatal child abuse. However, more recent studies indicate that mothers were responsible for the fewest number of child abuse cases. Bergman and colleagues (1986) concluded that fathers and the mother's boyfriend were the most common perpetrators in severe child abuse cases resulting in permanent injury or even death (Starling et al., 1995). Unfortunately, although women were found less likely to be the perpetrator of abuse, the number of fatal child abuse cases committed by women was equal to that committed by males (Starling et al., 1995).

There are a number of risk factors for becoming a perpetrator of child abuse. Poverty is the most frequently and persistently noted risk factor for child abuse (Bethea, 1999; Duhaime et al., 1998). Other societal factors include inaccessible and unaffordable health care, fragmented social services and lack of support from extended families and communities (Bethea, 1999; Duhaime et al., 1998; Lacey, 1998). Parents who were abused as children are more likely than other parents to abuse their own children (Bethea, 1999; Starling et al., 1995). Characteristics of the parent that increase the risk of child abuse include psychiatric impairments, substance abuse issues, emotional immaturity (i.e., teenage parents), poor coping skills, and poor self-esteem (Bethea, 1999; Lacey, 1998). Single parents are at greater risk for abusing their children as are those who are socially isolated, have a child younger than 18 months of age already present in the home, those who have a child with a disability or born prematurely or at a low birth weight, or the child is the result of an unwanted pregnancy (Bethea, 1999; National Committee on Child Abuse and Neglect, 1993-94). Risk for abuse also increases if another sibling has previously been reported to child protective services for suspected abuse (Bethea, 1999). No differences have been found in the incidence of child abuse in rural versus urban settings (Bethea, 1999).

There is a relationship between unemployment and physical abuse of children. It is not known whether this occurs because of increased psychological stress, or an increased number of hours an individual who is potentially abusive spends with a child (Krugman, Lenherr, Betz & Fryer, 1986). A study conducted by Krugman et al. (1986) in Colorado found that when unemployment was at a peak there were more reported cases of child physical abuse, contrary to when employment was high. During 1982 when unemployment in Colorado was at a peak, there were four deaths reported from the result of child abuse and three were in the homes of the unemployed (Krugman et al., 1986).

Elder Abuse

The dynamics of, and factors causing, elder abuse can be numerous and complex. There are many reasons for elder abuse; it may be the result of a strained caregiver, a long-standing history of abuse, or a combination of factors. Several theories of causation have been explored, but no consistent profile has been established for the elder at risk for abuse (Lachs & Fulmer, 1993). However, there are certain characteristics that increase the risk for becoming an abuser. These include: (1) being a spouse, (2) being the primary caregiver, (3) living with the abused, (4) disregard for frailty of the elder, (5) presence of personal problems, (6) dementia or confusion, (7) lack of experience caring for or being around the elderly, (8) mean spiritedness, being hypercritical of the elder, or showing tendencies to blame the elder, and (9) unrealistic expectations of the elder's abilities (Ferguson & Beck, 1983; Henton, Cate & Emery, 1984; Lachs & Pillemer, 1995; Larue, 1992; Pillemer & Finkelhor, 1988; U.S. Congress, 1990).

LEGAL AND ETHICAL IMPLICATIONS FOR THE OCCUPATIONAL THERAPIST

An occupational therapist is required to act on reported abuse according to state laws. Beginning in January of 1994, California became the first state to require doctors and nurses who treat battered women to notify police. Any licensed health practitioner must notify police as soon as possible and file a written report within 72 hours (Fehrenbacher, 1995). If a professional lives in a state that does not require the report of suspected domestic violence, the American Bar Association recommends providing referral numbers and lists of community resources to clients. A resource list and/or referral numbers can either be handed directly to the client or can be made available in discreet places such as bathrooms or private treatment rooms. Suggested numbers to be included in the list are: (1) local crisis lines, (2) local domestic violence shelters, (3) sexual assault crisis centers, (4) hospitals and medical centers, (5) victim advocacy programs, (6) individual and group counseling services, (7) legal services, (8) parenting classes, (9) counseling services for children who have witnessed or experienced abuse, (10) elder abuse referrals, (11) multilingual service programs and any other relevant information (American Bar Association, 2000).

When dealing with suspected elder abuse or abuse of a person with a disability, all states have adopted some form of adult protective services law, enabling state agencies to offer remedies to victims of abuse. All 50 states have enacted legislation authorizing the provision of adult protective services in cases of elder abuse. Generally, these laws establish a system for reporting and investigation and for the provision of social services to those victimized. In most jurisdictions, these laws also pertain to abused adults who have a disability/vulnerability/impairment as defined by state law, not just older persons (National Center on Elder Abuse, 2000). The majority of states mandate the reporting of elder abuse; however, there are no penalties for not reporting. And, if abuse is proved, fewer than half of the state laws provide civil or criminal penalties for elder abuse (AARP, 2000). If there is reason to believe that an elder is being abused, a professional should contact the local Department on Aging or Center for Independent Living or Adult Protective Services for the proper reporting procedure.

It is mandatory to report child abuse and neglect in all 50 states. Each state has passed some form of mandatory reporting law in order to qualify for funding under the Child Abuse Prevention and Treatment Act. All states require certain professionals to report suspected abuse: health care providers, facilities, mental health care providers, teachers, social workers, day care providers, and law enforcement personnel. Twenty states have broad statutes requiring "any person" to report (The Committee on Child Abuse and Neglect, 1997).

CONCLUSION

This article presented the scope and breadth of violence in the lives of individuals in the United States. Many of these individuals have the potential to be treated by occupational therapists who must understand their situations. Definitions of child, domestic and elder abuse have been presented with the hope of increasing occupational therapists' ability to identify victims in their practice. The risks of being abused and the effects of abuse were illustrated across the lifespan. Finally, the legal and ethical implications for the occupational therapist were presented to guide each therapist in his or her decision-making around reporting and intervening in the lives of domestic abuse survivors. It is the responsibility of each and every occupational therapist to understand the effects of violence on functioning and to educate him- or herself on appropriate procedures of intervention.

REFERENCES

Abbott, J., Johnson, R., Koziol-McLain, J., & Lowenstein, S. (1995). Domestic violence against women: Incidence and prevalence in an emergency department population. *Journal of the American Medical Association, 273*(22), 1763-1767.

American Association for Retired Persons web-page *http://www.aarp.org/ontheissues/ issueelderab.html*. Retrieved off of the World Wide Web on June 19, 2000.

American Bar Association (2000). Multidisciplinary responses to domestic violence at *www.abanet.org/domviol/mrdv/cando.html*. Retrieved off of the World Wide Web on June 19, 2000.

American Medical Association (1992). American medical association diagnostic and treatment guidelines on domestic violence. *Archives of Family Medicine, 1*, 39-47.

American Medical Association (2000). Diagnostic and treatment guidelines on mental health effects of family violence at *www.ama-assn.org/public/releases/assault/ fv-guide.htm*. Retrieved off of the World Wide Web on July 10, 2000.

Belsky, J. & Vondra, J. in Cicchetti & Carlson (Eds.) (1989). *Child Maltreatment: Theory and research on the causes and consequences of child abuse and neglect*. Cambridge University Press: New York, New York.

Bergman, A., Larsen, R., & Mueller, B. (1986). Changing spectrum of serious child abuse. *Pediatrics, 77*, 113-116.

Berkley Planning Associates web-page *http://www.bpacal.com/pressrel.html*. Retrieved off of the World Wide Web on August 31, 1999.

Bethea, L. (1999). Primary prevention of child abuse. *American Family Physician, 59*(6), 1577-1585.

Britton, H. (1998). Prenatal screening for child abuse and neglect. *Clinics in Perinatology, 25*(2), 453-460.

Butler, R. (1999, March). Warning signs of elder abuse. *Geriatrics, 54*(3), 3-4.

Centers for Disease Control and Prevention (1993). Emergency department response to domestic violence. *Morbidity and Mortality Weekly Report, 42*(32), 617-620.

Chicago Women's Health Risk Study at a Glance (2000). Illinois Criminal Justice Information Authority: Chicago, IL.

Council on Ethical and Judicial Affairs, American Medical Association (1992). Physicians and domestic violence: Ethical considerations. *Journal of the American Medical Association, 267*(23), 3190-3193.

Dearwater, S., Coben, J., Campbell, J., Nah, G., Glass, N., McLoughlin, E., & Bekemeier, B. (1998). Prevalence of intimate partner abuse in women treated at community hospital emergency departments. *Journal of the American Medical Association, 280*(5), 433-438.

Duhaime, A., Christian, C., Rorke, L., & Zummerman, R. (1998). Non-accidental head injury in infants: "The shaken baby syndrome." *The New England Journal of Medicine, 338*(25), 1822-1829.

Elliott, B.A. & Johnson, M.M.P. (1995). Domestic violence in a primary care setting. *Archives of Family Medicine, 4,* 113-119.

Fehrenbacher, G. (1995). California institutes abuse reporting law. *The Standard Times* at *www.s-t.com/projects/DomVio/californialaw.HTML.* Retrieved off of the World Wide Web on June 19, 2000.

Ferguson, D. & Beck, C. (1983, September/October). H.A.L.F.–A tool to assess elder abuse within the family. *Geriatric Nursing,* 301-314.

Ferris, L.E. (1994). Canadian family physicians' and general practitioners' perceptions of their effectiveness in identifying and treating wife abuse. *Medical Care, 32*(12), 1163-1172.

Fulmer, T. & O'Malley, T. (1987). *Inadequate care of the elderly: A health care perspective on abuse and neglect.* Springer Publishing: New York, New York.

Gerlock, A. (1999). Health impact of domestic violence. *Issues in Mental Health Nursing, 20,* 373-385.

Gin, N.E., Rucker, L., Frayne, S., Cypan, R., & Hubbell, F.A. (1991). Prevalence of domestic violence among patients in three ambulatory care internal medicine clinics. *Journal of General Internal Medicine, 6*(4), 317-322.

Goldberg, W.G. & Tomlanovich, M.C. (1984). Domestic violence victims in the emergency department. *Journal of the American Medical Association, 251,* 3259-3264.

Gondolf, E. (1988). Who are those guys? Toward a behavioral typology of batterers. *Violence and Victims, 2,* 187-204.

Gremillion, D.H. & Kanof, E.P. (1996). Overcoming barriers to physician involvement in identifying and referring victims of domestic violence. *Annals of Emergency Medicine, 27*(6), 769-773.

Hasselkus, B. (1991). Ethical dilemmas in family caregiving for the elderly: Implications for occupational therapy. *American Journal of Occupational Therapy, 45,* 206-212.

Healy, K., Smith, C., & O'Sullivan, C. (1998). Batterer intervention: Program approaches and criminal justice strategies. U.S. Department of Justice. *http://www.ncjrs.org/txtfiles/168638.txt.* Retrieved off of the World Wide Web on July 17, 2000.

Henton, J., Cate, R., & Emery, B. (1984). The dependent elderly: Targets for abuse. In W.H. Quinn & G.A. Hughston (Eds.), *Independent aging: Family and social system perspectives.* Gaithersburg, MD: Aspen Publications.

Hoff, L. (1992). Battered women: Understanding identification and assessment. *Journal of the American Academy of Nurse Practitioners, 4*(4), 148-155.

Holtz, H. & Furniss, K.K. (1993). The health care provider's role in domestic violence. *Trends in Health Care, Law & Ethics, 8*(2), 47-51.

Illinois Domestic Violence Act of 1986, P.A. 82-621, §101.

Johnson, T. (1991). Elder mistreatment: Deciding who is at risk. Westport, CT: Greenwood Press.

Johnston, J., Adams, R., & Helfrich, C. (2001). Knowledge and Attitudes of Occupational Therapy Practitioners Regarding Wife Abuse. *Occupational Therapy in Mental Health, 16*(3/4), 35-52.

Keller, L. (1996). Invisible victims: Battered women in psychiatric and medical emergency rooms. *Bulletin of the Menninger Clinic, 60*(1), 1-21.

King, M.C. & Ryan, J. (1989). Abused women: Dispelling myths and encouraging intervention. *Nurse Practitioner, 14*(5), 47-58.

Kosberg, J. (1988). Preventing elder abuse: Identification of high-risk factors to placement decisions. *Gerontologist, 28*, 43-50.

Koss, M. (1993). The impact of crime victimization on women's medical use. *Journal of Women's Health, 2*(1), 67-72.

Krugman, R., Lenherr, M., Betz, L., & Fryer, G. (1986). The relationship between unemployment and physical abuse of children. *Child Abuse and Neglect, 10*, 415-418.

Kurtz, P., Hick-Coolick, A., Jarvis, S. & Kurtz, G. (1996, June). Assessment of abuse in runaway and homeless youth. *Child and Youth Care Forum, 25*(3), 183-194.

Kurz, D. (1987). Emergency department responses to battered women: Resistance to medicalization. *Social Problems, 34*(1), 69-76.

Lacey, M. (1993). Patterns of abuse in the home. *Home Care Provider, 3*(6), 319-323.

Lachs, M. & Fulmer, T. (1993). Recognizing elder abuse and neglect. *Clinics in Geriatric Medicine, 9*(3), 665-675.

Lachs, M. & Pillemer, K. (1995). Abuse and neglect of elderly persons. *The New England Journal of Medicine, 332*(7), 437-443.

Lachs, M., Williams, C., O'Brien, S., Pillemer, K., & Charlston, M. (1998). The mortality of elder abuse. *Journal of the American Medical Association, 280*(5), 428-432.

Lafata, M. & Helfrich, C. (2001). The Occupational Therapy Elder Abuse Checklist. *Occupational Therapy in Mental Health, 16*(3/4), 141-161.

Larue, G. (1992). *Geroethics.* Prometheus Books: Buffalo, NY.

Massachusetts Coalition of Battered Women Service Groups and Children's Working Group (1995). *The children of domestic violence.*

Moss, V.A. & Taylor, W.K. (1991). Domestic violence: Identification, assessment, intervention. *AORN Journal, 53*(5), 1158-1164.

National Center on Elder Abuse at the American Public Human Services Association (1998). The National Elder Abuse Incidence Study; Final Report September 1998. *www.aoa.dhhs.gov/abuse/report/default.html.*

National Center on Elder Abuse (2000). Elder abuse laws: Information about laws related to elder abuse. *http://www.gwjapan.com/NCEA.* Retrieved off of the World Wide Web on June 21, 2000.

Nelms, B. (1994). Domestic violence: Children are victims too! *Journal of Pediatric Health Care. 8*(5), 201-202.

Neufield, B. (1996). SAFE questions: Overcoming barriers to the detection of domestic violence. *American Family Physician, 53*(8), 2575-2580.

Nosek, M. & Howland, C. (1998). Electronic resources for those working to end violence against women. *http://vaw.umn.edu/Vawnet/disab.html.* Retrieved off of the World Wide Web on August 31, 1999.

Olds, D., Henderson, C., Kitzman, H., & Cole, R. (1995). Effects of prenatal and infancy nurse home visitation surveillance of child maltreatment. *Pediatrics, 95*(3), 365-372.

Osofsky, J. (1995). Children who witness domestic violence: The invisible victims. *Social Policy Report Society for Research in Child Development, 9*(3).

Pascal, S. (1999). Save initiates SBS prevention program. *Pennsylvania Medicine, 102*(4), 19.

Peterson, L. & Brown, D. (1994). Integrating child injury and abuse-neglect research: Common histories, etiologies, and solutions. *Psychological Bulletin, 116,* 291-298.

Pillemer, K. & Finkelhor, D. (1988). The prevalence of elder abuse: A random sample survey. *Gerontologist, 28,* 51-57.

Quillian, J.P. (1996). Screening for spousal or partner abuse in a community health setting. *Journal of the American Academy of Nurse Practitioners, 8*(4), 155-160.

Quinn, M. & Tomita, S. (1986). *Elder abuse and neglect: Causes, diagnosis and intervention strategies.* New York, New York: Springer.

Randall, T. (1990). Domestic violence intervention calls for more than treating injuries. *Journal of the American Medical Association, 264,* 939-940.

Rath, G.D., Jarratt, L.G., & Leonardson, G. (1989). Rates of domestic violence against adult women by men partners. *Journal of the American Board of Family Practice, 2*(4), 227-233.

Reiss, A.J. & Roth, J.A. (1993). Panel on the understanding and control of violent behavior. Committee on Law and Justice, Commission on Behavioral and Social Sciences and Education, National Research Council. Washington, DC: National Academy Press.

Rivers-Moore, B. Disabled women's network for the national clearinghouse on family violence. *http://hwcweb.hwc.ca/hppb/familyviolence/html/womendiseng.html.* Retrieved off of the World Wide Web on August 31, 1999.

Rodriguez, M.A., Quiroga, S.S., & Bauer, H.M. (1996). Breaking the silence: Battered women's perspectives on medical care. *Archives of Family Medicine, 5,* 153-158.

Rosenberg, M.L. & Mercy, M.A. (1991). *Violence in America.* New York: Oxford University Press.

Russell, M. (1995). Piercing the veil of silence: Domestic violence and disability. *New Mobility,* 44-55.

Sassetti, M. (1993). Domestic Violence. *Primary Care, 20,* 289-305.

Stark, E. & Flitcraft, A. (1996). *Women at risk: Domestic violence and women's health.* Thousand Oaks, CA: Sage Publications.

Starling, S., Holden, J., & Jenny, C. (1995). Abusive head trauma. The relationship of perpetrators to their victims. *Pediatrics, 95*(2), 259-262.

Sugg, N.K. & Inui, T. (1992). Primary care physician's response to domestic violence. *Journal of the American Medical Association, 267*(23), 3157-3160.

Swagerty, D., Takahashi, P., & Evans, J. (1999). Elder mistreatment. *American Family Physician, 59*(10), 2804-2808.

The Committee on Child Abuse and Neglect (1997). Shaken baby syndrome: Inflicted cerebral trauma. *Delaware Medical Journal, 69*(7), 365-70.

Thormaehlen, D. & Bass-Feld, E. (1994). Children: The secondary victims of domestic violence. *Maryland Medical Journal, 43*(4).

U.S. Congress, House Select Committee on Aging (1990). Elder Abuse: A decade of shame and inaction. Washington, DC: U.S. Government Printing Office.

U.S. Department of Justice (1994, March). *Selected findings from the Bureau of Justice statistics: Elderly crime victims–National Crime Victimization Survey,* NCJ-147002. Washington, DC: Bureau of Justice Statistics, Office of Justice Programs.

U.S. Department of Justice (1997, April). *National crime victimization survey: Changes in criminal victimization,* NCJ-162032. Washington DC: Bureau of Justice Statistics.

U.S. Department of Justice (1997-98). Responding to victims with disabilities. *http://www.ojp.usdoj.gov/ovc/assist/nvaa/supp/t-ch21-12.htm.* Retrieved off of the World Wide Web on August 31, 1999.

Walens, D., Dickie, V., Tomlinson, J., Raynor, O., Wittman, P., & Kannenberg, K. (1995). *Mental health SIS education task force report.* American Occupational Therapy Association: Bethesda, MD.

Walker, L.E. (1994). *The battered woman syndrome.* New York: Springer.

Knowledge and Attitudes
of Occupational Therapy Practitioners
Regarding Wife Abuse

Jennifer L. Johnston, MS, OTR/L
Ralph Adams, MS, OTR/L
Christine A. Helfrich, PhD, OTR/L

SUMMARY. The purpose of this study was to determine if occupational therapists possess the ability to identify wife abuse by measuring their knowledge and attitudes about such abuse. A sample of 202 occupational therapists answered an average of 65% of knowledge questions correctly. Respondents were found to have empathic attitudes towards wife abuse and its victims, but were only slightly positive about the role occupational therapy should play in the identification of wife abuse. Knowledge and attitudes regarding wife abuse and the role of occupational therapy in its identification were all found to be significantly positively correlated. *[Article copies available for a fee from The Haworth Document Delivery Service: 1-800-342-9678. E-mail address: <getinfo@haworthpressinc.com> Website: <http://www.Haworth Press.com> © 2001 by The Haworth Press, Inc. All rights reserved.]*

KEYWORDS. Occupational therapist's knowledge, occupational therapist's attitudes, domestic violence

Jennifer L. Johnston is an Occupational Therapist (E-Mail: *c_j_johnston@email.msn. com*).

Ralph Adams is in Occupational Therapy, North Park University, 3225 W. Foster Avenue, Chicago, IL 60625-4895 (E-Mail: *radams@northpark.edu*).

Christine A. Helfrich is Assistant Professor, Department of Occupational Therapy, University of Illinois at Chicago, 1919 W. Taylor Street (M/C 811), Chicago, IL 60612 (E-mail: *Helfrich@uic.edu*).

This article was completed in partial fulfillment of a Masters of Science Degree in Occupational Therapy from Rush University in Chicago, Il.

For questions pertaining to this article, please direct all correspondence to Dr. Christine Helfrich.

[Haworth co-indexing entry note]: "Knowledge and Attitudes of Occupational Therapy Practitioners Regarding Wife Abuse." Johnston, Jennifer L., Ralph Adams, and Christine A. Helfrich. Co-published simultaneously in *Occupational Therapy in Mental Health* (The Haworth Press, Inc.) Vol. 16, No. 3/4, 2001, pp. 35-52; and: *Domestic Abuse Across the Lifespan: The Role of Occupational Therapy* (ed: Christine A. Helfrich) The Haworth Press, Inc., 2001, pp. 35-52. Single or multiple copies of this article are available for a fee from The Haworth Document Delivery Service [1-800-342-9678, 9:00 a.m. - 5:00 p.m. (EST). E-mail address: getinfo@haworthpressinc.com].

35

INTRODUCTION

Although the problem of woman abuse has been in existence for centuries, it was not until the 1970s that specific services were created to address the needs of the enormous population of women being battered (Davis, Hagen, & Early, 1994). At that time, shelters were opened; support groups were developed; and local, state, and national coalitions and agencies were formed (Davis, Hagen, & Early, 1994). To date, nothing has been sufficient in addressing the problem as the number of battered women continues to grow (Davis, Hagen, & Early, 1994). Women living in the United States are still more likely to be victimized by a current or previous partner than by all other assailants combined, whether through assault, rape, battery, or homicide (Council on Ethical and Judicial Affairs, 1992). Accurate demographic information is difficult to determine because much of the abuse is hidden and unreported; thus, incidence and prevalence rates of wife abuse are certainly undercounted (Isaac & Prothrow-Stith, 1997). However, in the United States alone, at least 2 million women are assaulted by their partners each year (American Medical Association, 1992), resulting in a reported total annual health care cost of approximately $44,393,700 (Moss & Taylor, 1991).

The American Medical Association (1992) defines "domestic violence" as a pattern of coercive control which may include repeated physical battering, psychological abuse, sexual assault, isolation, deprivation, and intimidation by a person who is either currently or was formerly intimately involved with the victim. Abuse is typically repeated and tends to escalate in both frequency and severity over time. The batterer often dominates and controls the woman through means such as restricting her access to food, clothing, money, social interaction, transportation, health care, or employment (American Medical Association, 1992). It is currently estimated that at least one abusive episode will occur in 33-50% of spousal and partner relationships (Russell, 1995). Pregnancy is considered to be a particularly high risk time for women as this is often the period when violence either begins or significantly escalates (Stark & Flitcraft, 1996). Approximately 23% of obstetric patients are involved in an abusive relationship (American Medical Association, 1992; Stark & Flitcraft, 1996). At even greater risk are those women having some type of disability. Eighty-five percent of them will be abused at some time (Nevada Network Against Domestic Violence, 1995). Abuse crosses all racial, socioeconomic, age, religious, and marital statuses (Stark & Flitcraft, 1996); thus, predicting abuse is often difficult. Considerable research on wife abuse has been conducted within the emergency care, primary care, and social service professions, but it is difficult to compare the results due to the variability in defining terms such as "battered," "abused," and "intimate partner." Researchers also employ various terms to describe the general phenomena, including "domestic violence," "family violence," "spouse abuse," and "partner abuse," but, as discussed by Yam (1995), these terms fail to reveal the gender and power issues which are at the heart of the problem in the majority of violent homes within the United States. Thus, the term "wife abuse" will be used throughout this study and is defined as any act which is intended to physically or emotionally harm that is taken against a woman by her male partner regardless of the current legal or domiciliary status of their relationship.

Research has shown that women typically will not voluntarily reveal the presence of abuse to their health care providers and most of these health care professionals do not ask about or address the battering either. This phenomenon has been referred to as "the unspoken agreement" between abused women and the rest of society (Rodriguez, Quiroga, & Bauer, 1996). However, a study conducted by Rodriguez, Quiroga, and Bauer (1996) found that nearly two-thirds of abused women want practitioners to ask directly about abuse. In this same study, 69% of abused women stated that they felt their health care providers should have a more thorough understanding of the psychological and social problems associated with wife abuse. Many abused women are negatively impacted by practitioners who simply treat the signs and symptoms of the abuse without directly asking about or addressing the underlying problem of domestic violence (Rodriguez et al., 1996).

C. Everett Koop demonstrated the critical nature of the problem when he recommended in 1986 that all health care professionals should be trained in the identification and intervention of domestic violence situations (Surgeon General's Workshop, 1986). However, recent studies conducted by various health professionals have found that the majority of practitioners still fail to recognize the presence of abuse and that even when it is identified, the degree to which providers offer therapeutic responses varies significantly. Of 1,521 health care professionals in six disciplines who completed a questionnaire regarding domestic violence, two-thirds were found to have no education on wife abuse. Of the six disciplines, only psychologists and social workers were identified as commonly suspecting abuse, and significant numbers of all professionals did not regard themselves as being responsible for intervening in cases of domestic violence (Tilden, Schmidt, Limandri, Chiodo, Garland, & Loveless, 1994).

Women who are abused often suffer from physical disabilities, psychosocial dysfunction, or both as a result of the violence. Abused women have suffered a significant blow to their sense of empowerment and self-esteem which affects their occupational performance (Gleason, 1993; Stark & Flitcraft, 1996). Furthermore, skills which may have been adaptive while in the abusive relationship, such as compliance, may not be adaptive if the woman chooses to leave the relationship (Gleason, 1993). Occupational therapy professionals are not only equipped with the skills necessary to address many of the physical manifestations secondary to the abuse, but they are also prepared to help these women develop adaptive coping skills, an internal locus of control, effective problem solving abilities, and improved communication skills. Nahmias and Froehlich (1993) argue that the prevalence of abuse compels all occupational therapy professionals to learn about the needs of abuse victims and to explore their personal feelings regarding abuse so they can employ treatment strategies which will provide victims with the opportunity to heal. Because wife abuse is so prevalent and crosses all demographic lines, it is likely that any occupational therapy practitioner who treats women will treat someone who is or was abused. Occupational therapy can play a critical role in the treatment of wife abuse victims. Due to the often intimate nature of the treatment occupational therapy practitioners provide and the duration of many of their patient relationships, these practitioners may be positioned to learn about aspects of their patients' personal relationships of which their physicians have not been informed. However, unless occupational therapy professionals are provided with at least a basic knowledge regarding the prevalence, indicators, and common sequelae of wife abuse, they may lack the ability to recognize cases of abuse within their patient population. In addition, if occupational therapy professionals do not hold appropriate therapeutic attitudes toward both abuse and the victims of it, such knowledge is not likely to be utilized effectively in the identification of violent relationships.

PURPOSE

The purpose of this study was to determine if occupational therapy professionals possess the ability to identify cases of wife abuse among their patient population. Ability, as defined in *Webster's Ninth New Collegiate Dictionary* (1986), is the "physical, mental, or legal power to perform" or a "natural talent or acquired proficiency" and was assessed in this study by measuring occupational therapy practitioners' knowledge and attitudes about wife abuse. This study did not attempt to uncover whether occupational therapy practitioners are actually using this ability to recognize and respond to cases of abuse, but merely whether they have the requisite skills to recognize abusive relationships. This study also explored what factors influence occupational therapy practitioners' ability to identify women as victims of wife abuse.

METHODS

This non-experimental quantitative study was conducted via a cross-sectional survey design using a mailed questionnaire. This approach allowed for efficiency of both time and economy while simultaneously providing information regarding the knowledge and attitudes that the more general population of occupational therapy professionals in the United States hold regarding wife abuse. Surveys are particularly well suited for assessing knowledge and attitudes because questionnaires measure what individuals *think* is true rather than what may actually *be* true. Questionnaires also allow measurement of both the prevalence and intensity of particular attitudes and beliefs and the differences in those attitudes and beliefs across various demographic groupings (Weisberg, Krosnick, & Bowen, 1996). Furthermore, due to the sensitive and potentially personal nature of the topic covered in this study, a mailed questionnaire allowed anonymity which likely improved the participation rate and decreased the threat to validity caused by pressure to provide socially desirable responses.

Population and Sample Selection

The population for this study included registered occupational therapists and certified occupational therapy assistants because both are likely to encounter abused women in their treatment sessions and are thus in a position to identify cases of domestic violence. The sample was randomly generated from the target population of practitioners who were current members of the American Occupational Therapy Association (AOTA) and who lived within the United States at the time of this study. AOTA randomly generated a list of practitioners from this target population and provided one set of mailing labels for the selected members to the investigator. The labels were used to mail 350 survey packets which included the cover letter, the questionnaire, and a self-addressed stamped envelope. All questionnaires returned within one month of the posted date were included in the study's results.

Instrumentation

Although a small number of questions were based on the work of Tilden et al. (1994), the majority of the instrument for this study was constructed using self-designed questions based on current literature regarding wife abuse. An expert in both domestic violence and occupational therapy was involved in the questionnaire development in order to improve the content validity of the instrument. To ensure consistent coding and analysis of data, all questions were written in a closed-ended format.

A pilot survey was conducted. A questionnaire and cover letter were distributed to 15 anonymous individuals in order to gain feedback. Pilot participants reported that the questionnaire was easy to understand and felt that the format and layout of the instrument were clear; therefore, no substantive changes were made to the questionnaire's content or wording. The final instrument consisted of 69 items which were broken down into three subsets of questions. The first subset of items was designed to collect information about various factors which have been shown to be related to the knowledge and attitudes that professionals within other health care disciplines have about domestic violence in general. Respondents were asked to provide information regarding their age, gender, practice area, and years of experience because each of these has been shown in studies of health care professional disciplines to be related to assessment of, and intervention for, wife abuse (Easteal & Easteal, 1992; Ferris, 1994; Reid & Glasser, 1994; Saunders & Kindy, 1993; Tilden et al., 1994). An additional series of items was included to address personal experience with abuse. Previous studies indicate that personal experience with abuse may affect the response of professionals to such cases within their patient population (Cullinane, Alpert, & Freund, 1997; Gremillion & Kanof, 1992; King, 1988). Several questions were designed to assess the amount and type of education regarding wife abuse each respondent has received as previous studies demonstrate that each of these factors impacts the identification rate of abuse (Campbell, Pliska, Taylor, & Sheridan, 1994; Reid & Glasser, 1997; Tilden et al., 1994; Yam, 1995). Respondents also were asked whether they feel adequately prepared to deal with suspected abuse. Studies have shown that even among those professionals who have received some education about wife abuse, many still do not feel they are equipped to address the issue with their patients (Reid & Glasser, 1997).

The next subset of questions was designed to assess the knowledge of the respondents regarding wife abuse; thus, the summary score of these questions was expected to present a basic picture of the general awareness that occupational therapy practitioners have about wife abuse. Some items addressed facts about abuse such as risk factors, batterer characteristics, and common reasons for staying in an abusive relationship. Some items within the subset addressed common physical, emotional, and psychological indicators and sequelae of abuse.

The final subset of questionnaire items was constructed in a 5-point Likert scale format to allow measurement of the intensity of each belief or attitude presented. As recommended by Dillman (1978) when attempting to measure attitudes, multiple questions were written to measure some of the constructs in this section in order to reduce bias based on wording.

RESULTS

Of the 350 questionnaires which were mailed, 202 (58%) were coded and included in the statistical analysis. Participants were found to have a mode age range of 31 to 40 years (37%). Of the 202 participants, 187 (93%) were female and 15 (7%) were male, which is consistent with the demographics of the overall member population of the AOTA (American Occupational Therapy Association, 1998). Participants had a mean of 11 years of experience. The majority of respondents practice as registered occupational therapists (78%), while the remaining 22% practice as certified occupational therapy assistants. Similar to the overall membership of AOTA which is 90% Caucasian (American Occupational Therapy Association, 1998), the majority of respondents in this study reported their ethnicity as "White, Not Hispanic" (87%). The highest degree earned by the majority (57%) was at the baccalaureate level. Survey respondents worked most frequently in a practice area they considered to be "Physical Disabilities" (44%), and 51% reported working predominantly with older adults.

Several questions within the demographic section of the instrument were designed to determine respondents' personal experience with abuse. A large number (22%) reported having been abused at some time by a male partner, while 12% indicated that they had been abused as children. The majority of respondents (53%) reported that they personally know two or more women who had been abused by a male partner, with another 25% reporting they know one woman who had suffered such abuse. These abused women are known in a variety of contexts.

A number of questions were included to assess the amount and type of education respondents had received regarding wife abuse. Most respondents reported having received no education, either formally (65%) or clinically (76%), about wife abuse. For those participants who have had some type of education on the topic, the aspects of the problem which have been covered within that education and the sources of their information have varied significantly. Sixty-eight percent of the study's participants do not feel that they are adequately prepared to identify cases of wife abuse, and even more (70%) do not feel they are prepared to provide either interventions or referrals to women being abused.

Thirty-five of the instrument's questions were designed to assess participants' knowledge about wife abuse. Frequency distributions were determined for each individual question. Total and average scores were then calculated for each respondent's survey, thereby allowing measures of central tendency to be determined for the total sample. These descriptive statistics were calculated in order to determine what occupational therapy practitioners know about wife abuse. Participants, on average, responded correctly to only 65% of the knowledge questions. Translated into percentages, scores ranged between 17% and 91% of knowledge questions being answered correctly, with a mode of 69% and a standard deviation of 13%.

Eleven of the Likert-scale questions were designed to assess occupational therapy practitioners' attitudes regarding wife abuse and wife abuse victims. Each respondent's average wife abuse attitude score was calculated, thereby allowing an overall average score to be determined for the survey sample. Because Likert-scale responses were coded as "2," "1," "0," " − 1," or " − 2," the average wife abuse attitude score had a possible range of − 2.00 to 2.00, with 2.00 representing highly caring attitudes toward wife abuse and wife abuse victims. The mean average wife abuse attitude score for all survey respondents was 1.49, with a standard deviation of 0.39. In other words, practitioners' overall attitude toward wife abuse fell approximately halfway between "Agree" and "Somewhat Agree" on the Likert scale. The lowest average attitude score among the respondents was − 0.54, while the highest average attitude score was 2.00.

The remaining five Likert-scale questions were intended to assess attitudes of occupational therapy professionals regarding their perceived role in the identification of wife abuse. For these items, each participant's average role attitude was first calculated, thus allowing measures of central tendency to be run on these averages. The overall mean role attitude score was calculated to be 0.53, with a standard deviation of 0.83. This translates to slightly over halfway between "Uncertain" and "Somewhat Agree." The lowest average role attitude score among participants was − 1.80, and the highest average role attitude score was 2.00.

This study also explored the relationship between occupational therapy practitioners' knowledge about wife abuse and their attitudes concerning such abuse. To determine this relationship, Pearson correlation coefficients were calculated to assess the relationship between the summary scores of the three subsets of questionnaire items. This analysis revealed that the overall average knowledge scores and the participants' attitudes concerning domestic violence are significantly positively correlated ($r = .182$, $p = .009$). The relationship between attitudes regarding wife abuse and attitudes about the role occupational therapy plays in the identification process was found to be even more strongly positively correlated ($r = .275$, $p = .000$). Finally, the strongest positive correlation was found between the average knowledge scores and the attitudes respondents have regarding the profession's role in the identification of wife abuse ($r = .276$, $p = .000$). Thus, as knowledge about wife abuse increases, the attitudes which occupational therapy professionals hold regarding wife abuse victims and the role they play in the identification of abuse become more strongly positive.

Finally, this study explored what factors are significantly related to occupational therapy practitioners' knowledge and attitudes concerning wife abuse and their role in identifying wife abuse. For those factors which had only two possible values, t-tests were run to compare the means of the two groups. Factors having more than two possible values were evaluated using analysis of variance (ANOVA). The age of an occupational therapy professional was found to be significantly positively related to his or her attitude about the role of occupational therapy in identifying cases of wife abuse ($F(4,197) = 5.62$, $p = .0003$). Female occupational therapy professionals were found to have a significantly more empathic attitude toward wife abuse and wife abuse victims than their male counterparts ($t = 2.58$, $p = .021$). Being abused as a child appears to be significantly related to the amount of knowledge one has regarding wife abuse ($F(2,198) = 3.90$, $p = .022$). An occupational therapy practitioner's attitude regarding the role that the profession should play in the identification of wife abuse is significantly related to both the amount of formal education he or she has received regarding wife abuse ($F(3,198) = 2.87$, $p = .038$) and his or her amount of clinical education regarding wife abuse ($F(3,197) = 3.74$, $p = .012$).

DISCUSSION

Four hypotheses were proposed to be tested as part of this study's research. The first hypothesis was that occupational therapy professionals have insufficient knowledge about wife abuse to effectively identify cases within their patient populations. Although it is difficult to say what amount of knowledge is "sufficient," the results of this study have shown that, for the population tested, knowledge about wife abuse was not extensive. The average score for the set of knowledge questions was only 65%, meaning that these therapists could answer less than two-thirds of the questions correctly. Furthermore, these questions were all written in a closed-ended format that required no recall, but only recognition to answer correctly. This finding can be compared to that of Cullinane (1997), who found that first-year medical students were able to answer, on average, 70-80% of questions about wife abuse correctly on a similar instrument. Only 12% of these medical students answered less than 50% of questions correctly, while more than twice that percentage (25%) of the occupational therapy professionals surveyed in this study answered less than half of the knowledge questions correctly.

Perhaps the most important indicator as to whether these therapists have sufficient knowledge about wife abuse to identify cases of such abuse is their own perception of being inadequately prepared. Sixty-eight percent of respondents stated that they do not feel adequately prepared to make such identifications within their patient populations. This percentage is higher than that found with physicians, as only 14% of physicians reported feeling incapable of identifying and addressing wife abuse (Reid & Glasser, 1997). This perception of inadequacy is important because it may affect occupational therapy practitioners' confidence in following up any suspicions they may have of the presence of violence within their patients' personal relationships.

The second hypothesis that was formulated was that occupational therapy professionals have a low acceptance of wife abuse. This hypothesis was supported as evidenced by the average attitude scores of the survey sample regarding wife abuse and wife abuse victims. Of the 202 respondents, only one had an average attitude score below zero, indicating this therapist was accepting of violence towards women and nonaccepting of its victims. Additionally, one participant had an average score of exactly 0.00 meaning this respondent felt uncertain about wife abuse and its victims. The remaining 200 respondents all had positive attitude scores; however, 18 of them (9%) had a low positive score, meaning they may have had some acceptance of violence against women and were only slightly empathic toward its victims. The remaining 90% of respondents had an average score of 1.00 or better, meaning they do not accept violence towards women and they are empathic towards its victims.

The third proposed hypothesis was that occupational therapy practitioners have negative attitudes about their role in identifying wife abuse. This hypothesis was not supported in that the average role attitude score was not less than zero; however, the average was only slightly positive (0.53). Furthermore, 20%, or 1 in 5 therapists surveyed, did have negative attitudes about the role of occupational therapy in the identification of wife abuse. Respondents held particularly negative ideas about whether therapists should screen all female patients for abuse, with 41% of respondents either disagreeing or somewhat disagreeing with the concept of such screening.

The fourth and final hypothesis presented was that occupational therapy professionals who possess greater knowledge about wife abuse have more positive attitudes about both the victims and the profession's role in working with them. This hypothesis was supported as demonstrated by the comparative statistics which were run. A significant positive correlation exists between the three subsets of questions, demonstrating that as knowledge about wife abuse increases, attitudes about both wife abuse and the role of occupational therapy in identifying such abuse improve. This finding lends further support to the argument for promoting and expanding education on the topic of wife abuse, as such education is likely to not only improve knowledge about the topic but also the attitudes held about wife abuse, its victims, and the role of the profession in identifying such abuse.

In addition to supporting the majority of hypotheses which were developed, this study resulted in several other important findings. The lack of education regarding wife abuse among the occupational therapy practitioners participating in the study was one such finding. Not only did 65% report having received no formal education about the issue, another 25% stated that they had received only one to two hours of instruction on the topic. Therefore, only 10% had received three or more hours. This lack of education is meaningful given the finding that such education is significantly related to the attitude therapists have regarding the role of the profession in identifying wife abuse, and is only slightly less than significantly related to the general attitude of practitioners toward abuse and abuse victims. Several respondents indicated on their survey instruments that they had received some education about child and elder abuse, but none about wife abuse. An increase in attention to wife abuse is warranted given both the prevalence of wife abuse and the call over one decade ago by the Surgeon General to include information on wife abuse in all health care curricula (Surgeon General's Workshop, 1986).

Another interesting finding of this study is the percentage of respondents reporting experiences of past abuse. Of the 202 respondents included in the data analysis, 22% identified themselves as having been abused at some time by a male partner, and 12% stated that they had been abused as a child. Perhaps even more interesting than the prevalence rates is the fact that having been abused as a child was found to be significantly related to the knowledge level of occupational therapy professionals about wife abuse ($F(2,198) = 3.90$, $p = .022$), while having been abused as an adult by a male partner had no significant relationship with either knowledge or attitudes about wife abuse. In addition to the high number of respondents reporting direct personal experience with abuse, 78% of participants reported that they knew at least one woman who is or was abused. It is important to acknowledge the possibility that these numbers may not be representative of the greater population of occupational therapy professionals, as those with such personal experience may have been more likely to complete and return this study's instrument than those sampled who did not have any type of personal exposure to wife abuse. The prevalence rates found in this study do, however, correspond with rates reported by first-year medical students where 13% reported having been abused as children and 32% reported abuse as an adult (Cullinane et al., 1997).

Limitations of the Study

Because so little research has been conducted to date within the occupational therapy literature regarding wife abuse, this study was designed to allow exploration of the topic. The lack of existing research within the field required the researcher to develop a self-designed questionnaire which did not have established validity or reliability. An expert in both domestic violence and occupational therapy was enlisted to help ensure as much content validity as possible, but it is certainly possible that this instrument did not elicit exactly the information it was intended to elicit.

Those individuals to whom a survey packet was sent who chose to respond were obviously self-selected and thus present a bias that could not be avoided when using a mailed questionnaire. This self-selection helped to ensure the anonymity of respondents, but is likely to have at least somewhat biased the sample. Practitioners with particularly poor knowledge about wife abuse may not have chosen to return their survey instruments because they were embarrassed or uncomfortable with how little they knew, regardless of the promised anonymity. The personal and sensitive nature of the material covered in this survey also may have encouraged respondents to choose what they felt were socially desirable responses. There is no way of ensuring that at least some respondents were not truthful in reporting their attitudes, although efforts were made to reduce this possibility. Based on these limitations, it is difficult to make any generalizations based on the results of this study to the broader population of occupational therapy professionals. It is only possible to state that these results would be applicable to a population which is highly similar to that studied here.

Implications for Occupational Therapy Practice

Although the majority of this study's respondents reported having received neither formal education (65%) nor clinical education (76%) about wife abuse, occupational therapy may not be that different from other health professions in this lack of training. A study of nurses revealed that 56% had not received any education regarding wife abuse (Limandri & Tilden, 1996). Clark, McKenna, and Jewel (1996) surveyed physical therapists about their recognition of battered women. These researchers found that only 8% of their study's participants had received any information on wife abuse in their education. Respondents in this survey indicated only slightly more training within their professional academic programs. Of the 202 respondents in this study, only 16% reported having their occupational therapy program provide any information regarding wife abuse. Not only are occupational therapy programs not including significant information on this issue, but other professional sources are not filling this gap. Only 13% of respondents reported that they had received information regarding wife abuse in their continuing education courses, and only 21% had received information about the topic from work colleagues. Since the time of Clark et al.'s study (1996), the American Physical Therapy Association (APTA) (1997) has instituted practice guidelines for the recognition and care of victims of domestic violence. Although it is not known whether this publication has resulted in improved identification of wife abuse by physical therapists, it is encouraging that the APTA has recognized its profession's need for information regarding work with this important population.

The current lack of education within the occupational therapy profession suggests that a similar commitment from the American Occupational Therapy Association (AOTA) is necessary to move the profession forward in its commitment to this important health and social issue. This commitment should include a call to academic programs to expand their curricula to include instruction on wife abuse, and more continuing education courses should be offered which address this issue. Many professional organizations, including the American Physical Therapy Association (1997), the American Academy of Family Physicians (1994), and the American Medical Association (1992), have made a commitment to the fight against abuse by issuing either guidelines or position papers about domestic violence. Unfortunately, as of this time, the American Occupational Therapy Association still has not issued any such documents. The issues on which a professional organization chooses to assume a position define to its members what the organization sees as the profession's values and purposes, thereby influencing what practitioners within that profession recognize and address with their patients. If the occupational therapy profession intends to adhere to its core values and to treat its patients holistically, then wife abuse should be addressed at not only the individual level, but at the organizational level as well.

As one respondent noted on her questionnaire, there is "no point in addressing other functional needs when the most basic needs of safety and self-esteem are not being met." Research within other disciplines has shown that women typically will not reveal that they are being abused if they are not asked (Rodriguez, Quiroga, & Bauer, 1996). If occupational therapy practitioners are not screening all female patients for abuse because they do not have the knowledge and attitudes needed to suspect abuse, it is entirely likely that they are failing to recognize the presence of abuse in many of their patients. Therefore, they may be falling into the same trap as many physicians of treating the signs and symptoms of abuse without addressing the underlying issue (Campbell et al., 1994).

To avoid making this mistake, occupational therapy professionals can employ a few basic concepts in their assessment and treatment of their patients. Practitioners can commit to consistently utilizing two important themes from the profession's theory, namely, treating the whole person and individualizing treatment. In order to do so, it is important that practitioners use interactive reasoning in collaborating with their patients. As described by Mattingly and Fleming (1994), occupational therapists "find themselves constantly confronted with the interpretive task of translating between their way of seeing and the patients.' If the goals that the therapists pursue are too far afield from the patients' perceptions of their functional needs, therapy is likely to be stalled" (p. 179). It is incumbent upon therapists to try to understand what an abused woman sees as her reality and how that reality affects her ability to function so that the practitioner and the woman can work together to develop possible therapeutic approaches.

For those women who are not comfortable with immediately revealing that they are or were being abused, it is especially important that practitioners utilize therapeutic use of self in their patient interactions. Occupational therapy professionals should strive to develop a context of safety, trust, and caring with their patients in order to promote open communication. The intimacy and duration of the relationships that occupational therapists often have with their patients are conducive to building such a relationship, and may thus result in the patient revealing many aspects of her home life and intimate relationship that she has been unwilling or unable to reveal to anyone else. In order to provide the most help to their patients, occupational therapists should be prepared to deal with such information if and when it is revealed.

CONCLUSION

The purpose of this study was to determine if occupational therapy professionals have the ability to identify cases of wife abuse among their patient populations. The occupational therapy professionals surveyed in this study did not possess extensive knowledge about wife abuse, correctly answering only 65% of questions which addressed facts about wife abuse such as risk factors, batterer characteristics, and common indicators and sequelae of abuse. Respondents, on average, were found to have fairly caring attitudes regarding wife abuse and its victims; however, they did not have correspondingly strong positive attitudes about the role of occupational therapy in the identification of wife abuse. In fact, 20% of all respondents held a negative attitude about the role of the profession in identifying wife abuse victims. Sixty-eight percent of the survey respondents stated they do not feel adequately prepared to make such identifications. Given these findings regarding both the knowledge and attitudes of the practitioners surveyed in this study, it does not appear that occupational therapy professionals currently possess the ability to identify victims of wife abuse within their patient populations. As both sets of attitudes were found to be positively correlated with knowledge about wife abuse, significant improvements in both knowledge and attitudes about wife abuse, and ultimately the ability to identify cases of wife abuse, may be possible if changes are made to include curricula regarding wife abuse within occupational therapy academic programs.

REFERENCES

American Academy of Family Physicians (1994). Family violence: An AAFP white paper. *American Family Physician, 50*(8), 1636-1646.

American Medical Association (1992). American Medical Association Diagnostic and Treatment Guidelines on Domestic Violence. *Archives of Family Medicine, 1*, 39-47.

American Occupational Therapy Association (1998, March). [Preliminary information from the member files]. Unpublished raw data.

American Physical Therapy Association (1997). *Guidelines for recognizing and providing care for victims of domestic violence.* Alexandria, VA: American Physical Therapy Association.

Campbell, J.C., Pliska, M.J., Taylor, W., & Sheridan, D. (1994). Battered women's experiences in the emergency department. *Journal of Emergency Nursing, 20*(4), 280-288.

Clark, T.J., McKenna, L.S., & Jewell, M.J. (1996). Physical therapists' recognition of battered women in clinical settings. *Physical Therapy, 76*(1), 12-18.

Council on Ethical and Judicial Affairs, American Medical Association (1992). Physicians and domestic violence: Ethical considerations. *Journal of the American Medical Association, 267*(23), 3190-3193.

Cullinane, P.M., Alpert, E.J., & Freund, K.M. (1997). First-year medical students' knowledge of, attitudes toward, and personal histories of family violence. *Academic Medicine, 72*(1), 48-50.

Davis, L.V., Hagen, J.L., & Early, T.J. (1994). Social services for battered women: Are they adequate, accessible, and appropriate? *Social Work, 39*(6), 695-704.

Dillman, D.A. (1978). *Mail and telephone surveys.* New York: John Wiley & Sons.

Easteal, P.W., & Easteal, S. (1992). Attitudes and practices of doctors toward spouse assault victims: An Australian study. *Violence & Victims, 7*(3), 217-228.

Ferris, L.E. (1994). Canadian family physicians' and general practitioners' perceptions of their effectiveness in identifying and treating wife abuse. *Medical Care, 32*(12), 1163-1172.

Gleason, W.J. (1993). Mental disorders in battered women: An empirical study. *Violence & Victims, 8*(1), 53-68.

Gremillion, D.H., & Kanof, E.P. (1996). Overcoming barriers to physician involvement in identifying and referring victims of domestic violence. *Annals of Emergency Medicine, 27*(6), 769-773.

Isaac, N.E., & Prothrow-Stith, D. (1997). Violence. In K.M. Allen & J.M. Phillips (Eds.), *Women's health across the lifespan: A comprehensive perspective* (pp. 439-453). Philadelphia, PA: Lippincott.

King, M.C. (1988). *Helping battered women: An examination of the relationship between nurses' education and experience and their preferred models of helping.* Ann Arbor, MI: UMI.

Limandri, B.J., & Tilden, V.P. (1996). Nurses' reasoning in the assessment of family violence. *Image: Journal of Nursing Scholarship, 28*(3), 247-252.

Mattingly, C., & Fleming, M.H. (1994). *Clinical reasoning: Forms of inquiry in a therapeutic practice.* Philadelphia: F.A. Davis Company.

Mish, F.C. et al. (Eds.) (1986). *Webster's ninth new collegiate dictionary.* Springfield, MA: Merriam-Webster Inc.

Moss, V.A., & Taylor, W.K. (1991). Domestic violence: Identification, assessment, intervention. *AORN Journal, 53*(5), 1158-1164.

Nahmias, R., & Froehlich, J. (1993). Women's mental health: Implications for occupational therapy. *American Journal of Occupational Therapy, 47*(1), 35-41.

Nevada Network Against Domestic Violence (1995, Summer). *Network News,* pp. 1, 4-5.

Reid, S.A., & Glasser, M. (1997). Primary care physicians' recognition of and attitudes toward domestic violence. *Academic Medicine, 72*(1), 51-53.

Rodriguez, M.A., Quiroga, S.S., & Bauer, H.M. (1996). Breaking the silence: Battered women's perspectives on medical care. *Archives of Family Medicine, 5,* 153-158.

Russell, M. (1995). Piercing the veil of silence: Domestic violence and disability. *New Mobility,* 44-55.

Saunders, D.G., & Kindy, P. (1993). Predictors of physicians' responses to woman abuse: The role of gender, background, and brief training. *Journal of General Internal Medicine, 8,* 606-609.

Stark, E., & Flitcraft, A. (1996). *Women at risk: Domestic violence and women's health.* Thousand Oaks, CA: Sage Publications.

Surgeon General's Workshop on Violence and Public Health Report (1986). Washington, DC: U.S. Department of Health and Human Services.

Tilden, V.P., Schmidt, T.A., Limandri, B.J., Chiodo, G.T., Garland, M.J., & Loveless, P.A. (1994). Factors that influence clinicians' assessment and management of family violence. *American Journal of Public Health, 84*(4), 628-633.

Weisberg, H.F., Krosnick, J.A., & Bowen, B.D. (1996). *An introduction to survey research, polling, and data analysis* (3rd ed.). Thousand Oaks, CA: Sage Publications.

Yam, M. (1995). Wife abuse: Strategies for a therapeutic response. *Scholarly Inquiry for Nursing Practice: An International Journal, 9*(2), 147-158.

PART II

Occupational Therapy's Role with Victims of Domestic Violence: Assessment and Intervention

Christine A. Helfrich, PhD, OTR/L
Ann Aviles, OTR/L

SUMMARY. Occupational therapists encounter individuals who are victims of domestic violence in many different settings. The role of the occupational therapist with each client depends on that client's specific needs, the treatment setting, and the skills and beliefs of the therapist. This article presents a theoretical argument for why the occupational therapist should choose to be involved in the treatment of domestic violence. The Model of Human Occupation provides a framework for understanding functional issues related to domestic violence. Methods of assessment and treatment are presented using this model. A continuum

Christine A. Helfrich is Assistant Professor, Department of Occupational Therapy, University of Illinois at Chicago, 1919 W. Taylor Street (M/C 811), Chicago, IL 60612 (E-mail: *Helfrich@uic.edu*).

Ann Aviles is Research Assistant, Department of Occupational Therapy, University of Illinois at Chicago (E-mail: *aavile1@uic.edu*).

The authors would like to acknowledge students from the University of Illinois at Chicago Occupational Therapy Program for their contributions to the development of occupational therapy interventions for survivors of domestic violence.

[Haworth co-indexing entry note]: "Occupational Therapy's Role with Victims of Domestic Violence: Assessment and Intervention." Helfrich, Christine A., and Ann Aviles. Co-published simultaneously in *Occupational Therapy in Mental Health* (The Haworth Press, Inc.) Vol. 16, No. 3/4, 2001, pp. 53-70; and: *Domestic Abuse Across the Lifespan: The Role of Occupational Therapy* (ed: Christine A. Helfrich) The Haworth Press, Inc., 2001, pp. 53-70. Single or multiple copies of this article are available for a fee from The Haworth Document Delivery Service [1-800-342-9678, 9:00 a.m. - 5:00 p.m. (EST). E-mail address: getinfo@haworthpressinc.com].

of levels of involvement including referrals for resources or treatment, direct and indirect treatment and program consultation is offered. Each level is illustrated with case vignettes demonstrating the therapist's role. Issues related to the challenge of working in domestic violence and reasons that women may refuse intervention are also discussed. *[Article copies available for a fee from The Haworth Document Delivery Service: 1-800-342-9678. E-mail address: <getinfo@haworthpressinc.com> Website: <http://www.HaworthPress.com> © 2001 by The Haworth Press, Inc. All rights reserved.]*

KEYWORDS. Domestic violence, model of human occupation, assessment

INTRODUCTION

Occupational therapists work with victims of domestic violence in every setting in which they are employed. The occupational therapist may not always be aware that the client with whom she or he is working is also a victim of domestic violence. The likelihood that the client is or has experienced domestic violence is increased if the person has a disability. Being abused and having a disability is a double disadvantage for women. Their disability may prevent them from leaving abusive situations or their partners may inflict injury resulting in disability (McNamara & Brooker, 2000). In other words, the women may have had preexisting disabilities not caused by the abuser or they may have disabilities as a result of the abuse. According to the National Crime Victimization Survey, approximately three-fourths of all violent events (e.g., rapes and assaults) involve an intimate or relative (U.S. Dept. of Justice, 1994).

Persons who experience domestic violence and disability encounter difficulties related to their disability (e.g., physical and/or mental limitations), and issues associated with domestic violence such as problems of poverty and economic dependence. These characteristics (e.g., physical limitations, economic dependence) often force women to remain in abusive relationships. Further, the safety of these women is most threatened when they attempt to leave their abusive situations (Holtz & Furniss, 1993). This places women in the predicament of relying on their abuser to survive, while jeopardizing their physical and/or emotional well-being. This combination of characteristics associated with domestic violence and disability comprises a population in need of specific services.

While in abusive relationships, battered women rarely have the resources needed to live on their own and are often financially controlled and isolated by their batterers (Brandwein, 1999). A barrier to obtaining more personal independence for many women who are victims of domestic violence is a poor work history. Women who are able to work outside the home often have poor attendance due to injuries and stress (Brandwein, 1999). In addition, they may be required to give their paycheck directly to their abuser who controls the finances. Thus, women who seek services geared toward creating more personal independence may increase their risk for further harm and/or further disability.

Financial issues are critical in a woman's decision to leave her abuser and whether she can become independent from him. It is also apparent that the pervasiveness of low-wage jobs limits the financial freedom that may prevent women from becoming homeless once they leave their abuser (Brandwein, 1999; Williams, 1998; Mullins, 1993). Because domestic violence shelters are often full and homeless shelters are reluctant to take victims of domestic violence, often the only choices for women are living on the streets or remaining with the abuser (Mullins, 1994). In New York City, after being sheltered, 31% of battered women returned to their batterers because they could not find low-income housing (Mullins, 1994). Emergency housing and support services for battered women may be the only real protection that society has to offer (Mullins, 1994). Shelters and other refuges for victims of domestic violence are ideal environments to address the skills that can prevent a woman from becoming homeless.

In addition to basic, traditional work skills, women often lack the life skills that are required to maintain a job and live independently (Helfrich, 1997). Women and the staff who worked with them in a transitional housing program identified difficulties with basic skills in budgeting, parenting, home management, stress management, anger management and other instrumental activities of daily living. However, there is little literature available that identifies or addresses the life skills required for victims of domestic violence to avoid becoming homeless. Occupational therapy has the potential to mitigate some of the life skill limitations that contribute to women becoming homeless.

In order for occupational therapists to assume their role with victims of domestic violence, the profession must begin to provide education and training regarding domestic violence. One of the primary reasons that occupational therapists do not address abuse with their clients is that they may not feel competent to do so (Johnston, Adams & Helfrich, 2001). How the therapist responds to a disclosure of domestic abuse has legal, ethical and practical implications. It is important for therapists to understand these implications in order to feel comfortable and competent. There are several levels on which to respond to the knowledge that a patient or client is a victim of domestic abuse, which range from providing referrals to other professionals to direct treatment of the abused woman.

The Cycle of Violence

In order to effectively evaluate an individual and respond to the results of that evaluation, the therapist must understand the range of experiences women have with their abusive partners. Lenore Walker (1979), in her classic text *The Battered Woman*, discusses this range of experiences as the Cycle of Violence. The Cycle of Violence has three phases.

- *Phase 1: Tension Building.* During this phase there is arguing, blaming, and tension in the relationship.
- *Phase 2: Battering.* This is the phase where the violence actually occurs. The violence may include physical violence such as slapping, choking, kicking, use of weapons, sexual abuse, and verbal threats and abuse.
- *Phase 3: Contrition.* This is the calm period after the abuse where the abuser denies the violence, apologizes, provides gifts or special treatment to the victim, and promises the abuse will not occur again.

This cycle represents a pattern of behavior that repeats itself. Each phase repeats, changing in relevant emphasis and severity over time. The Battering Phase will occur more frequently and the Phase of Contrition will be of shorter duration. In other words, as time goes on the battering increases in severity and occurs more frequently. The other phases may still occur but will lose their emphasis in the life of the relationship. This is why intervention with victims of domestic violence must occur. If the cycle is not interrupted, it is likely to eventually result in death (Chicago Women's Health Risk Study at a Glance, 2000). Intervention is most likely to be effective immediately after the Battering Phase. At that time the woman's defenses are down and she feels most vulnerable. She is most aware of the impact of violence on her ability to function. As she moves into the Contrition Phase she begins to feel stronger and more supported by her partner and may have more difficulty identifying the abuse as a problem.

ASSESSMENT

Occupational therapists routinely assess clients' safety in their current living situations. Safety assessments typically should include both physical safety and safety in the social environment. In the context of different practice settings, this safety assessment will take on different meaning. For instance, when the therapist is evaluating an individual's ability to return home independently after rehabilitation, the physical environment is always considered. Therapists routinely consider the availability of adapted bathroom equipment and grab bars, the placement of scatter rugs and whether or not a client can safely navigate in the kitchen. Likewise, a therapist who is working with a parent and child who live in a high crime community will assess the social environment for safety. Returning to an unsafe social environment will challenge the parent's ability to provide safe play opportunities for his/her child. While it may seem obvious to include family violence in a safety assessment, most therapists do not consider it part of a routine evaluation. Every occupational therapist should include the client's risk for domestic violence as part of a general safety assessment.

An ideal framework for assessing and understanding this population is The Model of Human Occupation (MOHO) (Kielhofner, 1995). This model was chosen because it permits persons to be viewed holistically and captures how the women function in their environment, while examining their roles, volition and habits. Table 1, "The Model of Human Occupation Applied to Domestic Violence," provides an out-

TABLE 1. The Model of Human Occupation Applied to Domestic Violence

MOHO SUBSYSTEMS	MOHO CONCEPTS	DOMESTIC VIOLENCE ISSUES Sample questions
ENVIRONMENT	A. Safety of Physical and Social Environment	1. Do you feel safe in your home? 2. Do you feel comfortable expressing your needs to people in your home?
	B. Physical and Social Supports	1. Does your environment support you doing what you need to do? 2. Are you able to rely on your significant other for support?
ROLES	A. Past, Current and Future Roles	1. Are you satisfied with your role(s)? 2. Are there past and/or future roles you would like to engage in?
	B. Impediments/Supports for Role Fulfillment	1. Is there someone or something that interferes with your ability to engage in desired roles? 2. Are there people or persons who support you pursuing desired roles?
HABITS	A. Daily Structure	1. Who determines how you structure your time? 2. Are you able to make spontaneous changes to your daily routine without consequences from others?
VOLITION	A. Sense of Internal Control	1. Do you feel in control of your actions? 2. Do you feel as though others dictate/control your actions?
	B. Belief/Appraisal of Skills	1. Do you feel confident in your ability to perform daily tasks? 2. Can you give me an example of something you do well?
	C. Values Related to Independence and Parenting	1. Do you feel confident in your ability to care for others? 2. Do you feel confident in your ability to care for yourself?
	D. Independent Interests	1. Are there activities you enjoy doing alone? 2. Are you able to engage in these activities?
MIND/BRAIN/ BODY	A. Physical, Emotional and Cognitive Functional Performance Skills	1. Do you feel you have the skills you need to live on your own? 2. Are there physical, emotional and/or cognitive limitations that affect your ability to get done what you need to day to day?
	B. Physical, Emotional and Cognitive Impediments to Leaving Abuser	1. Are there physical, emotional and/or cognitive limitations that inhibit you from leaving your abuser?

line of the domestic violence issues that relate to each subsystem of the model of human occupation.

Several tools based on The Model of Human Occupation provide a comprehensive assessment of women who are victims of domestic violence, including their self-care skills, communication/interaction skills, self-assessment skills and life history. The tools discussed in this article include:

1. The Occupational Performance History Interview (OPHI-II) (Kielhofner, Mallinson, Crawford, Nowak, Rigby, Henry, & Walens, 1998).
2. The Occupational Self-Assessment (OSA) (Baron, Kielhofner, Goldhammer, & Wolenski, 1999).
3. The Assessment of Motor and Process Skills (AMPS) (Fisher, 1999).
4. The Assessment of Communication and Interaction Skills (ACIS) (Forsyth, Salamy, Simon, & Kielhofner, 1998).

Occupational Performance History Interview-II (OPHI-II)

The OPHI-II is a semi-structured instrument that is administered in order to collect historical data on daily life experiences and on the impact of the environment on those experiences. The interviewer completes rating scales that explain the clients' values, self-esteem, lifestyle pattern, and environmental supports and constraints. The interview process takes one to two hours to complete.

This interview is comprehensive, allowing the interviewer to address past, current and future experiences. Although the tool allows a person to discuss the above areas, it does not speak to this population's specific experiences of being in an abusive relationship, and/or residing in an emergency shelter. However, because the OPHI-II is a life history narrative, it allows the therapist to address past and present domestic violence experiences. Obtaining this type of information can help the therapist identify life patterns and problem solving abilities.

Occupational Self-Assessment (OSA)

The OSA is a self-report, administered to measure the women's self-perception of their abilities, their satisfaction with their performance, and their views of the environment's effects on their performance. The OSA can be administered by the occupational therapist, or the client can choose to complete the assessment independently, and then review it with the occupational therapist. The OSA provides women the opportunity to self-reflect on their assets and limitations. It also affords women the opportunity to choose areas of personal importance that they would like to change. In many instances women are unable to make choices based on personal values due either to their abuser and/or the demands placed on them by the shelter. It also is an opportunity to discuss the impact of their environment on their ability to function.

The authors found it difficult to use the OSA with women who are concerned about potential declines in functioning in the future. For example, one of the women who completed the OSA reported "Taking care of myself" as a task she performs "very good" and is of "extreme importance"; however, this was an area she also identified as wanting to change. When questioned on her rationale for choosing to change how she is able to perform in relationship to this item, she summarized it by saying that this is an area she is able to do well currently due to the support of her environment. Conversely, she realizes that once she leaves the shelter environment, this is an area that may be difficult to maintain, due to the loss of structure and support provided through the shelter. This is indicative of a need to not only provide services for the women's current needs, but to also address their future service needs. Therefore, therapists need to closely examine skill areas being performed well and inquire as to whether or not women feel this may be difficult after leaving the shelter environment.

Assessment of Motor and Process Skills (AMPS)

The AMPS is an observation tool used to measure the motor and process skills of a person as routine tasks of personal significance are performed. This allows the observer to assess areas affected by a person's disability on their performance. Prior to observing two-three tasks, the client and the occupational therapist negotiate a task that the client performs routinely, while also ensuring that the task is not too easy or too difficult. The occupational therapist should aim for a "just right" challenge when selecting tasks. Once tasks are determined, the observer and client should discuss the specifics of the task to be performed in order to eliminate ambiguity as the client performs the task (e.g., deciding what type of bread, spread and meat the client will use to make a sandwich), and also where the tasks will be performed (e.g., common shelter living area vs. shelter resident's apartment).

Allowing the client to choose activities of personal significance that are performed routinely supports an increased sense of internal control. This is of great importance because many women who are in abusive situations do not have the opportunity to *choose* tasks that are important to them. Choosing activities also allows the women to feel in control of their actions. Often women in abusive relationships do not have control over the tasks they perform or even how they perform these tasks due to the controlling nature of the abuser. Permitting the woman to have control also increases her ability to make choices, introducing the woman to new and/or previous roles.

Therapists using this tool should be cognizant of the similarities and differences of the client's past, current and future environments. Women living in an emergency shelter are less likely to be familiar with their environment. They are put into situations where they cannot control with whom they are living (other shelter residents), or the neighborhood in which they reside. This environment may not be reflective of their previous and/or future environment. For example, a woman performed an AMPS task in the common living area of the shelter. This environment is reflective of her present living situation; however, it is not reflective of past and/or future environments, consequently, the assessment of her performance of the task may be inaccurate. Therapists should therefore be mindful in asking for information on the client's future social and physical environment.

The Assessment of Communication and Interaction Skills (ACIS)

The ACIS is an observational instrument. The ACIS assessment can be performed observing the client interacting with one person, in a group environment, or during 1:1 interactions with the client. The ACIS is used to analyze the behavior of a person when interacting in an individual and/or group setting. This tool allows the observer to assess areas such as social appropriateness, body language, and eye contact when interacting with one or more persons.

The ACIS allows a therapist the opportunity to evaluate social appropriateness (or inappropriateness) when a person interacts with others. However, the ACIS does not have a built-in mechanism for clarifying specific communication styles or mannerisms. This may be a crucial component for this population because their communication styles may have been influenced by previous interactions with their abuser. For example, one woman demonstrated an inability to make decisions regarding when and where the assessment process would take place. Although her score on the ACIS for "conforms" was high, her conformity (the ability to follow implicit and explicit social norms) made it difficult to schedule a meeting time and place. This behavior did not give the authors a good sense of what would be most convenient for her. Thus, her "over-conformative" behavior has implications for her ability to make her needs known to others. Conforming may have been an effective adaptation to her specific domestic violence situation; however, the same behavior may prove to be ineffective in many other situations.

During the assessment process, therapists who work with women who are victims of domestic violence need to appreciate the adaptive behaviors acquired by this population. Therapists should help women to identify these adaptive behaviors in order to assist them in recognizing their ability to change their domestic violence situation should this be of interest to the woman. In order to assess a woman's readiness to discuss her domestic violence situation, it is important to begin with global questions regarding her well-being and safety.

The assessment of domestic violence should begin with a general assessment of the client's safety in her home and living situation. After this assessment has been completed the following direct questions are recommended:

1. Do you feel safe at home?
2. Has there ever been a time when you did not feel safe at home?
3. Are there any situations in your life where you do not feel safe?
4. Is there anyone or anything that threatens your sense of safety?
5. Is anyone hurting you or your children?

These questions are recommended to ascertain if the client is currently in an abusive situation. The question, "Has there ever been a time when you did not feel safe at home?" refers to past abuse and is included here because of the repetitious nature of the cycle of violence (Walker, 1979).

These questions intentionally do not refer to "abuse" directly. The therapist should use clinical reasoning and careful judgment to follow up with the client on each of these questions. Simply inquiring, "Can you tell me about that?" will often open the door for discussion. Many clients will be relieved to have the opportunity to discuss their living situation with the therapist. At the point where the client has begun to trust the therapist, the therapist is in a better position to question her directly about her experiences with abuse. The therapist can then ask directly if the woman is being abused, what type of abuse is occurring, and how she feels about her situation. It is not uncommon for a woman to deny being abused and then minutes later to disclose that her partner "pushes her around" once in awhile. This does not necessarily mean that the woman is *deliberately* denying that she has been abused. Instead, it often indicates a lack of knowledge on her part that the behaviors she is describing are abusive. Women who were raised in abusive homes may not identify behaviors as abusive because they are experienced as normative to her. For these reasons, it is often not useful to initially ask a woman if she is being "abused." Focusing questions around being safe or being threatened may result in clearer answers.

In any area of practice the therapist must consider who else is present when questions regarding safety or abuse are being asked. Questions must *never* be asked in the presence of the person suspected of being the abuser. Asking questions in the presence of the abuser may place the woman at greater risk for further abuse. Even if she denies the abuse, the abuser may accuse her of leading the therapist to ask her about it. In some settings, such as home health care, finding a place to speak confidentially will be very difficult. The occupational therapist may need to be creative in order to create a context in which she can speak to the woman privately.

OCCUPATIONAL THERAPY INTERVENTION

Once the client discloses information that indicates the possibility of abuse, the therapist has an ethical obligation to respond in some manner. How the therapist chooses to respond will vary depending on state legal requirements, the treatment setting, theoretical beliefs and the therapist's skills and attitudes about his or her professional role. The response of the occupational therapist may occur in any of five ways: (1) following the legal requirement to report abuse, (2) initiating referral to resources or services, (3) offering direct treatment, (4) providing indirect services, or (5) utilizing program consultation. These types of intervention may be provided individually or as part of a collection of efforts by the therapist and other members of the health care team. Each type of intervention will be described with case vignettes to illustrate its application as occupational therapy.

Level 1: Report

Some states have mandatory reporting laws for domestic violence. Legal requirements range from the need to report any case of suspected abuse to those that only require reporting in cases where a deadly weapon was used. Each therapist should consult the Domestic Violence Act and Occupational Therapy Practice Act of his/her own state for details.

> *Illustration:* An occupational therapist practicing in home health observed a situation where she suspected abuse. When she reported her findings to the team, there was a mixed response. Some members of the team felt that the bruises she observed were simply from the woman's clumsiness and awkwardness adjusting to her new adaptive equipment. Other team members supported the OT's suspicion that the physical bruises, in combination with the client's vague statements about how poorly things were going at home, were indicative of possible abuse. In some states the therapist would be required to report these suspicions to the authorities.

Level 2: Referral

The occupational therapist may offer several types of referrals to a client who is either suspected of being a victim of abuse or who chooses to disclose her abuse. Referrals for domestic violence services include emergency housing, legal advice and assistance, and domestic violence counseling. Other types of referrals could include services for her children, psychotherapeutic counseling, or medical care.

The woman who is being abused is likely to be isolated from supportive friends and family either by the abuser or by having isolated herself to hide the abuse. In either case, she will need to rebuild a support system in order to heal and continue on with her life. The occupational therapist can refer her to support groups and agencies, which specialize in treating adult victims of domestic abuse. Most of these agencies also either provide services for children or will provide referrals for the children.

Clients may be relieved or pleased to receive referrals. They may also become very angry at the occupational therapist for suggesting that there is a domestic problem at home and refuse to accept any information. The Cycle of Violence (Walker, 1979) as a frame of reference can provide a way to understand the various ways that a woman might respond to the offer of a referral or the suggestion that she may benefit from assistance.

Whenever the therapist decides to offer information, the woman's safety must be given first consideration. Awareness of the form in which information is being provided and the environmental surroundings is critical. The information must be provided in a way that does not place the client at greater risk for abuse. Placing information in women's restrooms within the OT clinic area provides an opportunity for women to learn about domestic violence without their abuser's knowledge. Pamphlets and written information that could be found by the abuser are potentially dangerous to the woman. If her abuser finds domestic violence related literature on her person or with her belongings he may "punish" her for exposing his behavior to others. The occupational therapist must always respect a woman's judgment if she believes that accepting written information could be harmful to her.

Occupational therapists must be aware of local domestic violence crisis line numbers. Therapists should also be able to direct women or assist them to obtain basic information on safety and the availability of resources for her and her children. Therapists are encouraged to contact their local or state domestic violence coalitions for further information. The National Domestic Violence Hotline number is *1-800-799-SAFE (7233)*.

Level 3: Direct Treatment

Occupational therapy can offer many treatment options to a woman who is in an abusive situation. Occupational therapy, which directly addresses the issues of domestic abuse, may include the development of skills needed for successful role performance of desired roles, independent living skills, environmental adaptations, exploration of new roles, and educational, prevocational, or vocational treatment. Occupational therapists have an ethical responsibility to inform women of their treatment options. This would include options for maintaining the safety needed to pursue treatment.

The treatment setting and funding options available to the woman will influence provision of direct services. Occupational therapists who work in domestic violence settings are likely to work for the domestic violence agency and may be able to provide needed therapeutic services without seeking third party reimbursement. Hospital-based therapists are not as likely to have services paid by the agency. The issue of reimbursement should not prevent service provision. Instead, the hospital-based therapist may be more challenged to carefully identify the functional components which are most directly impacted by the domestic violence, and provide appropriate therapy services to address those issues.

> *Illustration:* A woman living in a transitional housing facility reported difficulty in effectively managing her anger, and expressed an interest in learning appropriate assertiveness techniques. She stated that she often keeps her anger bottled up and becomes depressed rather than letting others know how she feels. The OT in this setting worked with the client on learning to express herself and control her anger through assertiveness, and anger and stress management training.
>
> Another woman reported problems in organizing her daily routine, making it difficult to complete tasks throughout the day. The OT in this setting assisted her to develop and use a schedule/planner to organize her day. Together, they solved the problem of how to prioritize tasks throughout the day.

Level 4: Indirect Services

Occupational therapy may have a more effective role with victims of domestic violence through indirect service provision. Services are provided indirectly when the therapist works through non-occupational therapy staff to deliver services to clients. The therapist may offer training to staff to allow them to carry out recommended programs in the absence of the therapist. Because funding in domestic violence agencies is scarce, an occupational therapist may have more opportunities to provide services in this manner. The therapist who works in this type of setting may charge for consultation or may be there as a student-therapist completing a community-based field rotation under the direction of an occupational therapist. Occupational therapists can also provide in-service presentations to staff as part of a staff training program.

Illustration: Staff working with women in a transitional housing program reported that women were unable to follow through with their goals. The OT at the site worked with the staff to establish techniques for working with the women by educating the staff on how to help their clients establish realistic goals. This was accomplished by training the staff to break-up goals into multiple steps in order to make them more attainable. This assisted both staff and clients to see progress toward their goals which led to a higher percentage of clients following through and accomplishing their goals.

Level 5: Program Consultation

Occupational therapists also may provide program consultation in domestic violence programs. The occupational therapist's knowledge of systems, the environment, and activity analysis can be used for program consultation. The therapist may begin with a needs assessment and expand to a wide variety of roles. The therapist can collaborate with staff on program planning to develop life skills or community reintegration, to recommend participation in vocational and educational programs, or to expand an intake assessment process to include functional components. A relationship that begins as consultative may expand to include both additional areas of consultation or the development of a permanent position for an occupational therapist within an agency.

Illustration: A recent student project included a pilot needs assessment of 16 women that utilized the Occupational Self Assessment. The women identified stress management, finances, time management and opportunities to do things they valued as areas on which they needed to work. Through informal interview they also identified assertiveness/self-expression and goal setting as areas of need. The students used this information to create resource materials for staff that focused primarily on budgeting and stress management. The staff reported that the resource book was a useful tool. They expressed a desire to have more comprehensive information available to them to make informed decisions about programming.

REASONS WOMEN REFUSE INTERVENTION

Despite offering information or interventions to a woman, she may not accept it when it is offered. The refusal of assistance can be frustrating for occupational therapists; however, the therapist should not feel his/her efforts have been futile. The average woman leaves her abusive partner five to seven times before staying away (Russell, 1995). There are a variety of reasons that a woman may refuse assistance and choose to stay in, or return to, an abusive relationship. These include: economic pressure, belief he will change, fear of being harmed, no place to go, love, fear of being alone, concern for the children, guilt, concern for the abuser, and pressure by others (NiCarthy, 1982).

This range of experiences contributes to why the woman has difficulty leaving the relationship. It is important for the therapist to know that even if an intervention is initially refused, the intervention may still have an impact on the woman's life. She may remember the intervention or return to the information provided, weeks, months or years later when she is ready to accept it. Women have called crisis lines and arrived at emergency shelters with referrals from all types of sources (Helfrich, 1997). As information providers, occupational therapists cannot always know when a client will use the information provided.

CONCLUSION

Occupational therapists will work with victims of domestic violence in every setting. The role of the therapist in each case will be determined by the client's needs and the therapist's skill and attitude regarding domestic violence. This variability must change and it should become standard practice for occupational therapists to consider it ethically necessary for the domestic violence to be addressed. Education and role modeling will facilitate this change.

This article has provided a theoretically based outline of assessment and treatment procedures for the occupational therapist. Each occupational therapist is challenged and encouraged to pursue this information and acquire the essential knowledge to treat this critical population.

REFERENCES

Baron, K., Kielhofner, G., Goldhammer, V. & Wolenski, J. (1999). *A User's Manual for The Occupational Self Assessment.* The Model of Human Occupation Clearinghouse, Department of Occupational Therapy, Chicago, IL.

Brandwein, R.A. (1999). *Battered Women, Children and Welfare Reform.* Thousand Oaks, London, New Delhi: Sage Publications, Inc.

Chicago Women's Health Risk Study at a Glance (2000). Illinois Criminal Justice Information Authority, Chicago, IL.

Fisher, A. (1999). *Assessment of Motor and Process Skills, 3rd Ed.* Department of Occupational Therapy, Colorado State University. Fort Collins, CO: Three Star Press.

Forsyth, K., Salamy, Simon, & Kielhofner, G. (1998). *A User's Guide to The Assessment of Communication and Interaction Skills, version 4.* The Model of Human Occupation Clearinghouse, Department of Occupational Therapy, Chicago, IL.

Helfrich, C. (1997). Unpublished Dissertation Title: Homeless mothers experience of transitional housing: An ethnographic study. Ph.D. Public Health Sciences-Community Health, The University of Illinois at Chicago.

Holtz, H. & Furniss, K.K. (1993). The health care provider's role in domestic violence. *Trends in Health Care, Law & Ethics, 8(2),* 47-51.

Johnston, J.L., Adams, R. & Helfrich, C. (2001). Knowledge and attitudes of occupational therapy practitioners regarding wife abuse. *Occupational Therapy in Mental Health, 16(3/4),* 35-52.

Kielhofner, G. (1995). *The Model of Human Occupation: Theory and Application, 2nd Ed.* Baltimore: Williams & Wilkins.

Kielhofner, G., Mallinson, T., Crawford, C., Rigby, M., Henry, A., & Walens, D. (1998). *A User's Manual for The Occupational Performance History Interview-II,* The Model of Human Occupation Clearinghouse, Department of Occupational Therapy, Chicago, IL.

McNamara, J.R. & Brooker, D.J. (2000). The Abuse Disability Questionnaire: A new scale for assessing the consequences of partner abuse. *Journal of Interpersonal Violence, 15(2),* 170-183.

Mullins, G.P. (1994). The battered woman and homelessness. *Journal of Law and Policy, 3,* 237-255.

NiCarthy, G. (1982). *Getting Free: A Handbook for Women in Abusive Relationships.* Seattle, WA: The Seal Press.

Russell, M. (November, 1995). Piercing the veil of silence: Domestic violence and disability. *New Mobility,* 44-55.

U.S. Department of Justice (1994). *Selected Findings from the Bureau of Justice Statistics: Elderly Crime Victims–National Crime Victimization Survey,* March, NCJ-147002. Washington, DC: Bureau of Justice Statistics, Office of Justice Programs.

Walker, L. (1979). *The Battered Woman.* New York, NY: Harper & Row Publishers Inc.

Williams, J.C. (1998). Domestic violence and poverty: The narratives of homeless women. *Frontiers, 19,* 143-165.

Assessing Needs and Developing Interventions with New Populations: A Community Process of Collaboration

Deborah Walens, MHPE, OTR/L
Christine A. Helfrich, PhD, OTR/L
Ann Aviles, OTR/L
Lisa Horita, OTR/L

SUMMARY. The predominance of chronic and lifestyle-induced conditions has emphasized the need for greater access to health care in the community. A corresponding concern is educating practitioners so they are equipped to assume positions in the community at graduation. Lack of preparation to work in the community has led to reluctance on the part of practitioners to pursue positions in the community (Walens et al., 1998). However, the current climate of health care creates many opportunities for practitioners and educators who are willing to make a commitment to work collaboratively with agencies in the community for a common good. The purpose of this paper is to broaden understanding of community built practice by sharing a collaborative process in fieldwork

---

Deborah Walens is Clinical Assistant Professor, University of Illinois at Chicago, 1919 W. Taylor Street (M/C 811), Chicago, IL 60612 (E-mail: *dwalens@uic.edu*).

Christine A. Helfrich is Assistant Professor, Department of Occupational Therapy, University of Illinois, Chicago, IL (E-mail: *Helfrich@uic.edu*).

Ann Aviles is Research Assistant, Department of Occupational Therapy, University of Illinois, Chicago, IL (E-mail: *aavile1@uic.edu*).

Lisa Horita is Staff Occupational Therapist, Rausch Rehabilitation Services, Chicago, IL.

The authors of this article would like to thank the community agency and their students for the opportunity to learn first hand about the collaborative process as they implemented this program.

The authors would also like to thank the U. S. Department of Health and Human Services, Grant 1-D377 AH-00607-01 for support in the fieldwork Level II training.

[Haworth co-indexing entry note]: "Assessing Needs and Developing Interventions with New Populations: A Community Process of Collaboration." Walens, Deborah et al. Co-published simultaneously in *Occupational Therapy in Mental Health* (The Haworth Press, Inc.) Vol. 16, No. 3/4, 2001, pp. 71-95; and: *Domestic Abuse Across the Lifespan: The Role of Occupational Therapy* (ed: Christine A. Helfrich) The Haworth Press, Inc., 2001, pp. 71-95. Single or multiple copies of this article are available for a fee from The Haworth Document Delivery Service [1-800-342-9678, 9:00 a.m. - 5:00 p.m. (EST). E-mail address: getinfo@haworthpressinc.com].

education that was undertaken by faculty at the University of Illinois at Chicago. *[Article copies available for a fee from The Haworth Document Delivery Service: 1-800-342-9678. E-mail address: <getinfo@haworthpressinc. com> Website: <http://www.HaworthPress.com>* © *2001 by The Haworth Press, Inc. All rights reserved.]*

KEYWORDS. Community fieldwork, collaborative learning, collaborative supervision, domestic violence

THE NEED FOR COMMUNITY BUILT PRACTICE

The need for community built practice has become more evident, as health has become more central to containing the cost of illness, and patterns of mortality and morbidity have shifted from acute infectious disease to a predominance of chronic and lifestyle-induced conditions. Policy makers (Tresolini & Shugars, 1994; Shugars, O'Neil, & Bader, 1991; Soto, Berhrens, & Rosemont, 1990) have responded to this concern by emphasizing prevention and greater access to health care in the community. This has led to services moving outside their traditional medical settings and into the communities where people live and work. Although situated in the community, it is important to remember that models of community care have developed on a continuum. The continuum ranges from community-based practice which retains its medical focus by addressing the individual or family's immediate needs; in contrast, community built practice engages the community with its multiple dimensions, perspectives and relationships to build a practice that integrates diverse strategies and methods of practice (Walter, 1997, p. 69). Said another way, the scope of practice ranges from an expert or authoritarian model of practice to one that is community and family centered.

The need for practitioners to develop the skills and understanding of community practice in mental health was well documented in the 1995 *Mental Health Special Interest Section Education Task Force Report* (Walens et al.). As we begin the twenty-first century, occupational therapy educators and practitioners face challenges and opportunities to effectively prepare students for future practice in the community. As Kielhofner (1992) points out, the medical model has dominated practice beginning in the late 1940s and 1950s with the occupational therapy profession developing a strong affiliation with physicians and movement toward reductionism and then a mechanistic paradigm of practice. A call for a new paradigm in the 1960s and 1970s by Reilly and others was aimed at returning the central focus on occupation. With the focus on occupation the community becomes the ideal context for practice. As this paradigm has slowly evolved, education has maintained its strong alliance with the medical model and student-practitioners continue to have a major emphasis of their education in medical-based practice settings. A paucity of preparation to work in the community has led to reluctance on the part of practitioners to pursue jobs in the community (Walens et al., 1998); however, the current climate of health care creates many opportunities for practitioners and educators willing to make a commitment to work collaboratively with agencies in the community for a common good. Partnering with community agencies creates a win-win situation for all parties and when well done expands the context for occupational therapy practice. Prerequisite for entering the community is a mind set that values collaborative partnerships and emphasizes the identification, nurturing and celebration of community assets (Minkler, 1997, p. 6). As the context of practice shifts, preparation of faculty and students for successful community built partnerships will necessitate a change in the education process. As educators are traditionally schooled in a medical or expert model of practice, faculty will need to reconceptualize roles and functions to integrate essential aspects of community built practice. In order to do so, practitioners need to be aware of major differences between the two contexts of practice (found in Table 1).

PHASES OF COMMUNITY BUILDING

Critical to the process of developing a community partnership is understanding the need to invest time and make a commitment for the long-term. The essence of community built practice relies on being able to relate to the community as if you are a part of it. This requires having an understanding of the complexity of the system and working toward being less of an outsider. To this end faculty at the University of Illinois at Chicago have made a conscious decision to maintain ongoing relationships with community agencies by pursuing funding of faculty time. The purpose of this paper is to broaden understanding of a community built practice by sharing a collaborative process in

TABLE 1. Comparison of Hospital OT and Community OT

Aspect of Practice	Hospital	Community
Focus of practice	Individual patient	Population or person in context of community
Timeframe for service	Brief, short-term	Ongoing
Referent term	Patient	Client, resident, participant or consumer
Health is defined as	Absence of illness	Wellness, increased quality of life, or increased choice over one's well-being
Access	Limited opportunity to observe family relationships or other indicators of health	Multiple opportunities to observe family relationships and factors that impact health
Environment	Limited patient autonomy	Encourages family and community autonomy and control
Professional role	Expert	Collaborator
Roles	Defined with clear boundaries	Negotiated, blurred, often ambiguous
Supervision	Direct, line-of-site	Collaborative, consultative
Peer relationships	Limited to hospital personnel	Extends beyond agency and seeks to create synergies in the community.

Source: Adapted from B. Logan & C. Dawkins (1986). *Family-centered nursing in the community.* Menlo Park, CA: Addison-Wesley Publishing Co.

fieldwork education that was undertaken by faculty at the University of Illinois at Chicago.

This community collaboration occurred with a Comprehensive Domestic Violence Agency. The agency operates a transitional housing program for women and their children who had been victims of domestic violence. Within the transitional housing program was a day care center oriented toward meeting the needs of children which included the Head Start Program and a Before and After School Program. Additionally, the agency provided a Home Start Program, emergency shelter, an outreach program, police liaison program, and supported housing. Table 2 describes each of the children's programs, the focus of our initial involvement, and the types of services available.

An initial relationship developed in 1996, when the Department of Human Services funded an external evaluation of the demonstration Head Start program for homeless children operated by the agency. David Beer was the Principle Investigator and Christine Helfrich was the on-site evaluator. Helfrich's role was to conduct a qualitative evaluation comprised of action-research methods, which then gave the opportunity to provide input into program development at the agency. She was initially given entrée to the agency, but still needed to establish a trusting relationship; such that, staff was willing to provide necessary information and not feel threatened by her presence. Although sounding like common sense, the strategies used to build trust

TABLE 2. Descriptions of Agency Programs[1]

Program Name	Ages Served	Program Focus
Home Start	0 to 2 years	Home-based program using home visitors. In weekly home visits, children's development is assessed in an ongoing fashion, screening is done for medical disorders, depression, eating/sleeping disorders, and children are referred for appropriate services. In addition, mothers are taught how to provide appropriate stimulation for their infants.
Head Start	2 to 5 years	A center-based all-day program as mothers are required to work or be in work training with a typical Head Start curriculum integrating 2/3 homeless and 1/3 community children.
Before and After School Program	6 to 12 years	Provides support for moms so they can work or be enrolled in a training program. Provides children with breakfast and light meal after school, assistance getting ready for school and with homework, escort to and from school, structured and unstructured activities. In summer program expanded to all day.

[1]Source: From "Chicago Homeless Head Start Demonstration Project Evaluation Final Report: Evaluation of Ridgeland Enhanced Head Start Program for Transitional Housing Residents," by David W. Beer and Christine A. Helfrich, 1996, University of Illinois at Chicago, Department of Occupational Therapy.

may not be as commonly found in a medical milieu. Examples of strategies used to build trust included:

• Learning people's names and knowing how they personally wanted to be addressed.
• Eliminating professional jargon in verbal communication and incorporating terms used by the staff to discuss concerns about children.
• Being careful not to slip into an authority or expert role.
• Building opportunities in discussions to hear staff concerns.
• Picking topics to discuss that had been identified as important to staff.

The relationship with the community agency quickly developed and broadened to allow for the exploration and development of occupational therapy practice through a consultative model.

The purpose of the Head Start program evaluation was to demonstrate whether or not Head Start was effective in the lives of children. The program's effectiveness was measured by its ability to halt developmental delays and promote development in the children enrolled in the programs. At the time the evaluation began, the Head Start Program used the DIAL-R (Mardell-Czudnowski & Goldenberg, 1990) to assess and measure a child's development. This tool is based in the education literature and did not include psychosocial development.

The on-site evaluator, an occupational therapist, shared her concern that in a program where all of the children had witnessed violent and traumatic events, it was important to assess their psychosocial functioning. The lack of sensitivity of the DIAL-R to identify and measure deficits was also raised as a concern. With this finding it became important to identify a tool that could be administered by teachers with limited formal education about disability. It was also important to find a tool that was efficient to administer and easily interpreted. After a comprehensive review of the literature and consultation with a number of pediatric educators and clinicians, the First Step Screening Test for Evaluating Preschoolers (Miller, 1993) was identified. This tool was based on occupational therapy theory, but designed to be administered by a variety of disciplines, including teachers. The on-site evaluator completed several assessments with children who represented the range of functioning seen in the day care programs and presented these cases to staff to illustrate the utility of the tool.

In the role of on-site evaluator, opportunity arose in the context of giving feedback to educate the staff about occupational therapy. These discussions created occasions for sharing what an occupational therapist might contribute to the agency. Occupational therapy was introduced in a non-threatening manner as the on-site evaluator provided consultation regarding children who were of concern to the teachers. Those actions led staff to accept the use of the First Step. Introducing the First Step to teachers provided an opportunity for in-service education on child development and consultation with teachers on their skill development for administering the First Step. These formal relationships allowed informal introduction of other OT concepts to further explore and describe the potential role for OT in this setting.

A year after introducing the First Step to the staff, the idea of creating a fieldwork site for an occupational therapy student team (OTS team) was introduced to staff and subsequently supported by administration. Since the on-site evaluator had opportunities to both observe and hear staff concerns, the Before and After School Program serving children ages 6-12 years was identified as a priority for introducing occupational therapy students.

All stakeholders (administration, staff and parents) agreed the Before and After School Program had not received the same amount of attention as the Head Start based programs. During the time of the program evaluation the on-site evaluator's only involvement with the Before and After School Program had been to follow some of the children who had graduated from Head Start into the Before and After School Program. Once the need was identified, a proposal for creating a Level I fieldwork site was put forth to the staff. The proposal stated that if an OTS team was placed at the site, they could assist in completing a needs assessment of the Before and After School Program. This assessment could help the agency understand the concerns that teachers, administration and parents had with respect to the Before and After School Program. While completing the needs assessment the OTS team would also have an opportunity to begin providing some services to the children. The agency saw this as an opportunity to learn more about the needs of the children and to increase services for them on at least a temporary basis. They gave permission to bring three occupational therapy students for a Level I fieldwork, which is completed on a full-time basis for four weeks during the summer. This was at a time when the school children would be attending the Before and After School Program all day. Because the administration knew and trusted the on-site evaluator and were pleased with the impact she had had on the Head Start Program, they saw this as an opportunity not only to provide services but also to improve the programming of the Before and After School Program.

DEVELOPMENT OF A FIELDWORK SITE

Clarifying the Role of the Occupational Therapy Student Team

The development of the site for educating Fieldwork Level I OT students illustrates the ongoing collaborative relationship that was and continues to be maintained at the agency. While initial observations had led to some ideas about what OT could offer and where best to start, the teachers in the program were consulted to elicit their input on what would be the best use of the OTS team in the Before and After School Program. In an initial planning meeting two central questions were asked: (1) Are there areas that you would like to develop if you had more time or more staff to help you? (2) Are there certain times of the day when you have more difficulty managing the children or keeping them focused on the task you are trying to complete? Also, in order to continue to build trust, the on-site evaluator placed on the table the question, "What are some of your worries or concerns about having interns?" The consultant was aware that the agency had had psychology interns before and the experience was not positive for the teachers. The teachers responded by sharing that the psychology interns always pulled the students out of the classroom when they met with them and after the student returned to class there was no report to the teacher. Their lack of follow-up with the teachers created problems particularly when the discussion had upset the child. A decision was made in the meeting that the OTS team would work with the students in the classroom, and would provide ongoing feedback to the teachers about what they were doing and observing with the children by verbally reporting to the staff at the end of each day.

The teachers were also concerned as to how the OTS team would be oriented to the agency. A decision was made that the agency staff would conduct the orientation prior to the OTS team's arrival. This would create an opportunity for staff and the OTS team to begin to form a relationship. The final area that was covered in the planning meeting was a discussion of the OTS team's background and education. This discussion gave an opportunity to familiarize the teachers with the knowledge that students received on child development and behavioral issues often associated with children who have had exposure to domestic violence. This planning meeting facilitated the teachers having input into what the OTS team would be doing in their classroom and also made sure that the OTS team would be focusing on concerns of the teachers. Several areas were identified which were reframed in terms of what OT could offer. This provided further opportunity for education and collaboration. Together the on-site evaluator and the classroom teachers developed a preliminary plan for the OTS team. It was emphasized that this was *preliminary*, as everyone agreed the plan would be modified based on an ongoing dialogue between the teachers, the OTS team and UIC faculty supervisor.

Selecting the Occupational Therapy Student Team

From the academic side we wanted to make sure that the fieldwork experience went well. It was the first chance to introduce occupational therapy and an OTS team formally in this setting, and it was important to succeed in order to continue and expand the Department's involvement in the future. To that end, the academic fieldwork coordinator (AFC) at UIC and the on-site evaluator, who will now be referred to as the faculty supervisor, created a special application form for OT students who were interested in the site (refer to Table 3). OT students were asked to describe their motivation to complete fieldwork in the setting, identify learning styles, describe communication strengths and liabilities, clarify their desire to engage in a community fieldwork that used a collaborative learning model, and identify strategies employed when dealing with ambiguous roles. Applicants also attached a *Professional Behavior Self-Assessment* (Walens, 1997) to the application. The students were required to self-assess ten areas of professional behavior including: commitment to learn, interpersonal skills, communication skills, effective use of time and resources, use of construc-

TABLE 3. Personal Assessment for a Community Placement on Fieldwork Level I

PERSONAL ASSESSMENT FOR COMMUNITY PLACEMENT FOR FIELDWORK LEVEL I

1. Please explain your interest in this site.

2. The model of supervision for this site is a collaborative learning model. Describe what you expect your relationship will be with your peers and the supervising OTR during this fieldwork experience.

3. Please comment on your preferred learning style. Explain how you like to learn. Describe what creates a positive learning experience for you and what is more challenging.

4. Describe your leadership abilities and opportunities you have actively pursued to develop your leadership skills in the past 5 years.

5. Describe your communication abilities; discuss at least 2 or 3 skills you consider your strengths and 2 or 3 you are still developing.

6. Describe your usual response to situations where you are assuming an active leadership role and there is a lack of structure and ambiguity about your role.

7. List and describe volunteer or paid employment that you feel would enhance your ability to work at this agency. Identify your role in each of these experiences.

Attach a copy of your Professional Behavior Assessment.

---

tive feedback, problem-solving, professionalism, responsibility, critical thinking and stress management.

All applications were processed and coded by an assistant to remove personal identifiers. The faculty supervisor and AFC then completed a blind review of the applications. Applications were then prioritized to determine the appropriateness of each OTS for placement at the site. The faculty supervisor and AFC met to discuss the applications and any disagreement they had in determining the selection of three students to be placed at the agency. When differences in ratings occurred, discussion of the rationale used in rating the application followed and a consensus was developed to make a final decision.

Preparing the Occupational Therapy Student Team for a Community Placement

Three OT students were selected who had a strong interest in the placement and the necessary skills to work as a collaborative team. In the semester before fieldwork, the OT students completed coursework that focused on the development of skills necessary for effective collaboration including active listening skills, building and maintaining a climate of trust in the group, developing leadership and group member skills and conflict resolution. Additionally, they completed a psychosocial course with modules on domestic violence and attended an orientation provided by agency staff.

Our model of education and supervision for this fieldwork experience relied on collaboration and self-directed learning instead of a traditional apprenticeship model that is dependent on close direct supervision. The literature points out (Knowles, 1984; Martens, 1981; Wiley, 1983; Bruffee, 1987; Herge & Milbourne, 1999) that collaboration and self-directed learning fosters a social context for learning which is central to working effectively in the community while supporting independent and interdependent critical analysis, clinical reasoning and creative problem solving. As the community agency was a setting without an occupational therapist, it was then necessary for the on-site teacher/supervisor to serve as the specialist in the domain of understanding the operations of the program and the children at the agency while serving as a role model and resource to the OTS team. The faculty supervisor consulted with the OTS team and expected them to be self-directed in getting their needs met using a collaborative team approach to supervision. The anticipated outcome was that the OTS team would effectively develop competence in community practice and would develop collaborative relationships with each other and with staff in the agency.

Collaborative learning methods were chosen for a number of reasons. First, without an occupational therapist consistently at the agency the OTS team needed to be responsible not only for individual successes but the success of the team. If the team created a positive interdependence with individual accountability to the group, we believed the outcome would be successful. To assure the success of the group it was vital for each OTS to be self-directed in assessing individual needs and pursuing resources to meet those needs before asking for help from the on-site supervisor or contacting the faculty supervisor. To assist the students in developing these skills prior to arriving at the agency, each participated in coursework that had a major emphasis on collaborative learning. As discussed by Bruffee (1995), working together does not come naturally; it is something we learn how to do.

Clarifying Roles and Responsibilities

As there were multiple levels of collaborative supervision that took place during the fieldwork experience (see Table 4), it became important to clarify the roles and responsibilities for the OTS team, on-site teacher/supervisor, and off-site faculty supervisor.

Roles and responsibilities were clarified as follows:

On-Site Supervisor Responsibilities:

- Clarify arrival time, dress code, directions to the facility, and other logistical issues.
- Provide orientation to the facility, staff, policies, procedures, protocols for safety and precautions, documentation and record keeping.
- Give facility tour.
- Collaborate with faculty supervisor to determine assignment of children.
- Orient OTS team to facility communication systems.
- Provide information regarding the children.
- Provide feedback on interactions with children.
- Provide feedback on participation in the program, interactions with staff and professional behavior.
- Provide feedback on leadership in groups using feedback form.
- Collaborate with off-site faculty supervisor to give feedback on accuracy of observations documented in SOAP note.
- Be available as a resource for questions on program, policies, procedures, children/residents.
- Have a consistent daily check-in with the OTS team in morning or afternoon to plan and/or process.
- Meet formally once a week with student team to discuss issues and give feedback.
- Meet once a week with faculty supervisor and as needed during the week.
- Assign children to OTS after consultation with the faculty supervisor.
- Assign groups to OTS after consultation with the faculty supervisor.
- Clarify availability of resources at the facility for OTS use.

- Assist faculty supervisor in completing an evaluation of individual OTS performance.

Off-Site Faculty Supervisor Responsibilities:

- Meet with on-site supervisor prior to students arriving to plan fieldwork Level I experiences, discuss how OT students will work collaboratively and schedule regular meetings to discuss how the student team is working.
- Identify readings for OTS team.
- Meet weekly with OTS team to process experience.
- Schedule times for observing OTS team at facility.
- Collaborate with on-site supervisor in the review of weekly documentation and give feedback on occupational therapy reasoning.
- Give feedback to OTS on treatment/care plans for children.
- Review and give feedback to OTS on group write-ups.
- Collaborate with on-site supervisor to complete evaluation of student performance.
- Meet with student team prior to fieldwork to orient to readings, assignments, expectations and roles. Clarify schedule.
- Be available on an "as needed" basis for phone consultation to OTS.

Occupational Therapy Student Responsibilities:

1. After assignment to the agency, the OTS team will meet and determine who will contact the agency to:

- Confirm assignment with contact person.
- Clarify time of arrival on day one and hours expected to be present at the facility.
- Determine the dress code.
- Obtain directions to the agency.
- Clarify other logistics that arise in their meeting.

2. Prior to beginning the fieldwork experience:

- Meet with the faculty supervisor to clarify the supervisory schedule.

- Successfully complete course work on collaborative learning.
- Complete readings related to agency assignment.
- Familiarize self with assessment tools used at facility.

3. During orientation:

- Understand the program philosophy.
- Meet with on-site supervisor to go over schedule, define role within the agency, clarify expectations of experience.
- Review policies and procedures of the facility.
- Clarify questions regarding the role of the on-site supervisor and his/her supervisory style.
- Understand the safety procedures and precautions of the setting.
- Tour the facility.
- Understand the facility's system of communication both written and verbal.
- Understand admission criteria and procedures.
- Meet interdisciplinary staff and understand their roles.
- Understand family rights and guidelines for participating in the program.
- Know the community agencies used for referral.

4. During the fieldwork experience:

- Work together with the OTS team to problem-solve daily questions that arise before taking them to either the on-site or off-site supervisor. OTS team must therefore be able to differentiate between issues they can resolve, issues where they have limited knowledge and issues that require communication with a supervisor.
- Utilize journals for logging questions, concerns, and dilemmas for discussion with on-site and off-site supervisors.
- Take responsibility for meeting OTS team's needs and personal needs.
- Manage communication between on- and off-site supervisors.
- Work with a caseload of two to four children over the course of the fieldwork experience.
- Familiarize self with children through record review and introduce self to children.

- Review all group write-ups, documentation and care plans in OTS team meetings for feedback before turning in to the on-site or off-site supervisor.
- Complete weekly SOAP notes on all assigned children.
- Complete Group Activity Plan one day prior to leading a group.
- Complete all assignments in a timely manner.
- Modify behavior in response to feedback from OTS team and in response to on-site and off-site supervision.
- Provide feedback to peers on OTS team.

The OTS team served at the agency for four weeks, 40 hours per week. Their role was primarily as indirect service providers, but they also provided limited direct service. The off-site faculty supervisor was scheduled at the site about 10 hours each week and was available by phone. Students had contact with the off-site faculty supervisor most days either in person or by phone, and they also kept journals to communicate their feelings about the experience and their reactions to the process. Journals were collected regularly and the off-site supervisor responded to issues and concerns that surfaced. The journals provided a valuable means for communication on topics that may not have surfaced in face-to-face supervision but were critical to supporting the learning process for the OT students. The role of the off-site supervisor was to provide OT supervision and help the OTS team identify the occupational performance issues of the children they were assigned. Also, the off-site supervisor served as mediator between the OTS team and the agency staff when role conflicts occurred. The on-site teacher/supervisors provided important information on programs, policies, procedures, and details on assigned children. Students

TABLE 4. Types of Collaborative Supervision

• OT student to OT student collaboration
• Off-site faculty supervisor and OTS team collaboration
• Off-site faculty supervisor and on-site classroom teacher/supervisor collaboration
• On-site classroom teacher/supervisor and OTS team collaboration.

also had daily "check-ins" with the on-site teachers/supervisor in order to process information or concerns about a child.

The Academic Fieldwork Coordinator had a peripheral role once the OTS team began the fieldwork experience. She was available as a resource for students, but it was suggested that they use the resources of the team, the on-site supervisor and the off-site faculty supervisor before turning to the AFC for help. During the four-week experience, the OTS team also met with the AFC and 11 other students on Fieldwork Level I for two synthesis sessions which focused on debriefing of the experience, group problem-solving and case study presentations.

CHALLENGES IN DEVELOPING COMMUNITY FIELDWORK

Student Challenges

In order to understand both the challenges and benefits of the first year of the program, a two-hour interview was conducted with the OTS team. The interviewers, a physical therapist and research specialist in the college, were not directly involved with the fieldwork experience. The interview was transcribed and coded to identify themes that reflected the challenges and benefits of the experience. In hindsight, it would also have been helpful to conduct a formal interview of the teachers at the agency. The following information on the teachers' perspective reflects discussions the teachers had with the faculty supervisor.

There were a number of challenges during the first year of the program that created multiple learning opportunities for the OT students, faculty and the agency. Throughout the four weeks of fieldwork the OTS team struggled with its OT identity and often questioned if they were doing "real OT" as their experiences did not match those of other OT students who were placed in hospital-based Level I fieldwork. They seemed to miss the direct "hands-on" treatment. Direct treatment in this community-based experience was limited to assessing children who were more puzzling to the teachers. They used the First Step and the Children's Self Assessment of Occupational Functioning (Curtin & Baron, 1990) to assess the children while their major role was to provide consultation to the teachers. In retrospect, one student stated,

I think the way we helped most was doing the activity analysis and bringing new activities . . . we had books and tons of activities . . . these kids have anger issues, they have self-esteem issues, well what activity can we bring in that's going to make them feel better about themselves, it's (the activity that is) going to be able to allow them to deal with their inner issues. I think we got the gist of it towards the 3rd and 4th week when we were like really rolling.

The OTS team found the implementation of a consultative model demanding as they reasoned strategies for dealing with a number of issues in the classroom, i.e., anger management, self-esteem, age appropriate activities for children, learning to play cooperatively. Another student explained the challenges of working with classroom teachers, who were cooperative in turning over the class to them.

One activity that we did was playing house, they had a lot of clothes (at the agency) and . . . the teachers were more on the sidelines just watching . . . we did some role playing. . . . We tried to share information with the staff (about the activity). I'm not sure we included them enough in the activities. . . . I wished they had participated more because this was for (them) as well as for the children so they could use these ideas later on. . . . One positive thing is that they (the teachers) are very open to us coming in and sharing our ideas. . . . They were very open to what we had to give to their program.

As consultants to the teachers, the OTS team created an Activity File using a Group Planning Form (see Table 5), role modeled planning and implementation of activity groups and restructured the environment to support better behavioral outcomes with the children. Often suggestions made by the children were incorporated into activity plans. Another member of the OTS team remembered a successful activity plan and reflected on her level of active listening in working with the children.

The hat activity, it was one that we had taken from one of the student's (suggestions); he said something about wanting to make a hat out of newspaper . . . so we tried to take interests of theirs (the children) and put them into activities. I think he was really excited; that they are listening to me and they made this activity about something I wanted to do and I think he mentioned something (like) "well I just kind of said it" but he didn't expect anything would come of it.

Learning to trust one another and deal with team conflict was an ongoing part of supervision. There were a number of factors that contributed to this challenge: (1) the team had various levels of experience and comfort working with children; (2) the team had different communication styles; (3) there were differences in age–a 10 year range; (4) there were differences in preparation–two were bachelor level and one was a master's level student; (5) each student had a different rapport with the faculty supervisor given their relationship prior to the fieldwork experience; and (6) there were racial and ethnic differences that came forth in a setting where most staff and families were African-American. One of the students was Hispanic, one was Caucasian and one was Asian. When discussing the differences one student commented,

I didn't feel different, the kids obviously had not seen someone who is Asian before, there were a lot of curious questions.

While a second student shared,

. . . it was a little bit uncomfortable at first, but I got over that and it wasn't the children, I think it was more of working with the adults. . . . I'd never worked in a setting that was completely of a different (culture), I haven't worked in a setting where it was all African-American people and a culture that was low income. . . . I think it was an uncomfortable feeling that I imposed upon myself that I got over quick.

Faculty Supervisor Challenges

The faculty supervisor also experienced challenges, which needed to be addressed in a timely way. One of the first areas needing attention was setting limits on agency staff for using the OTS team as "extra help." This issue often presents a dilemma, as outsiders need to become a part of the community. It is important not to be perceived as aloof by refusing to pitch-in, but there is also an obligation on the part of the faculty supervisor to monitor the educational experiences of the

TABLE 5. Group Planning Form

GROUP PLANNING FORM
Name of activity _____
Date of planned activity _____
In planning a group clarify and elaborate on the following:
• Number of participants (clarify minimum and maximum)
• Materials needed (list all supplies needed)
• Environmental requirements/considerations (specify ideal environment, include precautions)
• Directions for activity and suggestions for presentation to children (be specific)
• Goals: (Consider all aspects–physical, emotional, cognitive, sensory, interpersonal) *On back of sheet list specific goals for targeted children*
• Anticipated problems or contraindications and solutions or modifications
• Group's response to activity/modifications to consider

students so that their needs are met. As an outsider one must also recognize the pay-offs of pitching-in and the opportunity it presents for community building.

A second challenge that developed for the faculty supervisor was the transition from her former role as on-site evaluator where she was working for the agency to the role of faculty supervisor with her allegiance split between the staff and the OTS team. She needed to be cognizant of the needs of both parties and to weigh who needed priority. An example was recognizing that on-site supervisors found it difficult to give objective feedback to the OTS team as the teachers felt as if they were "picking on" the OTS team if they gave negative feedback. This experience identified an important area of training for the on-site supervisors. One student who felt she would have learned more if negative feedback had been given all along raised the issue during the interview.

You don't know how other people are thinking until you actually ask them; the reason I say this is on the last day, we're sharing feedback and I got feedback from one of the teachers that was completely new to me and it was something that was a problem with the way I was interacting with the children, it was something that never even crossed my mind when I was there. . . . We always got . . . "everything's good," everything's good all the time, so on the last fieldwork evaluation, concerns came up that I never even knew existed.

Agency Challenges

In the community agency both staff and families experienced challenges with the implementation and presence of the OTS team. Staff initially felt threatened by the presence of outsiders in the classroom and needed to develop comfort and trust that their presence would not have a negative impact on them. Staff also felt threatened by the OTS team's professional knowledge even though they recognized that the OTS team had knowledge that the teachers did not have and that the OTS team didn't claim to know everything! Families experienced the OTS team as another intrusion to their privacy and schedule. As outsiders, the OTS team needed to earn their trust. This was additionally challenged by the fact that some families had had negative experiences with previous interns from another discipline.

THE BENEFITS OF COMMUNITY FIELDWORK

Student Benefits

The benefits of the experience in the first year clearly created a synergy that led to the growth of the fieldwork program. Of equal importance was the fact that the students found the experience to be as valuable as that of their counterparts who had completed hospital-based fieldwork. The major concern on the part of the students was "Will I be as prepared as other students who did a fieldwork in a medical setting?" The OTS team found they had many opportunities to develop clinical reasoning and also learned how to clearly define their role. When asked what it was like to be supervised by a non-OT and an OTR consultant one student answered,

I think if we would have had an OTR telling us "This is what you're here to do," I don't think we would have been as effective because it would have been more like a cookbook and we were able to bring in kind of our own ideas.

The OTS team also became skilled in teamwork, using multiple models of collaboration and being self-directed in finding and using resources. In discussing some of the skills they developed in class prior to Fieldwork Level I, one student reflected on being assertive in giving feedback to the teachers and with each other.

I don't think that was just for us to (be assertive with) the teachers, I think it was also within ourselves you know it's different, it's one thing to say, "you know blah, blah, blah, blah, blah," and it's another to have to stop and think . . . you have to be objective, cause we had to give each other feedback on some of the assessments. . . . You learned to be more professional.

Each OTS developed self-confidence and independence in flexibly assuming the role of a student-therapist in the setting and dealing with constantly changing schedules as well as the need to be flexible in scheduling groups and assessments. An equally important outcome was that each student had an appreciation for the lives of the children, families and staff of the agency. This was probably one of the most profound aspects of this experience. This quote is representative of what the team learned from some of the children who were victims of domestic violence,

I learned what it's like from their (the children's) perspective of going through transitional housing, it made everything just seem so real, you can only read so much out of a book, but when you hear it from their perspective and you see how they (children) interact with other children, I mean, it just, it opens your eyes.

Faculty Supervisor Benefits

A major advantage for the faculty supervisor was accomplishing more in the same amount of time with three student-therapists who completed needs assessments and helped gather data related to the children and the classrooms. The data gathered by the student-therapists was used in ongoing research projects. She also found that collaborative supervision was enjoyable and well suited to her personal style of letting students develop at their own pace and in their own directions.

Agency Benefits

The benefits for staff were identified as obtaining skills and resources that would improve the quality of the program they provided for the children. They viewed the OTS team as a valuable addition to the classroom both in terms of alleviating stress but also in their contributions of new and creative ideas for the children. The OTS team helped them appreciate the complexity of therapeutic activity and mutual respect developed through the collaborative process. This led to increased interest in having occupational therapy students in the future. The teachers also increased their confidence in supervising interns, which had broader application in the agency.

The children directly benefited from the additional services and given their positive comments to the OTS team, it was hypothesized that this experience had a positive effect on their development of skills. The increased trust demonstrated by the children led the agency to invite UIC students to return in the future.

OUTCOMES OF THE PROJECT

The Fieldwork Level I program in the first year was able to provide consultation on two major areas that were identified in the needs assessment (1) environmental modification and (2) activity analysis and therapeutic activity education. In the second year, two additional components were added. The OTS team began to administer the OT Psychosocial Assessment of Learning (Townsend et al., 2000) to the children and began conducting groups on conflict resolution with an emphasis on anger management skills.

Experiences with Fieldwork Level I informed the development of a longer Fieldwork Level II experience which was funded as part of an Allied Health Professions Project through U.S. Department of Health and Human Services, Grant #1-D377 AH-00607-01. This funded project allowed us to expand the team to include nutrition students and develop services for the mothers who are participating in a transitional housing program. A relationship that began with a contract for program evaluation developed into multiple opportunities to create new

OT practice areas, fieldwork experiences for students and a context for faculty scholarship in the community.

CONCLUSION

The faculty has learned that we can challenge the traditional methods of educating students and be successful. When working in the community we discovered proactive planning needs to be emphasized. Student preparation and selection are critical; you need to define the skills that students need to enter the setting and teach those skills prior to their arriving at the community agency. Building rapport with the agency staff, incorporating their ideas throughout the process and providing ongoing supportive consultation to the agency staff is key for the success of the program. Open and honest communication among all parties involved in the project is foundational to success.

One caution is a need for balance between the emphasis of peer collaboration and the role modeling by the OTR. Creating an environment where peers consistently discuss and problem-solve is not enough to meet the clinical reasoning needs of student-therapists. Regular interaction with an OTR (expert) role model is required so that the students' critical thinking is challenged and channeled beyond their limited perspectives. When educating student-therapists in the community, one needs to help them re-frame "real OT" and help them define their OT role in the setting. One of the myths of practice is that "real OT" constitutes providing "hands on" services (Walens et al., 1998). As professionals and educators, it is important to define occupational therapy also as consultation and indirect service with other non-OT professionals, para-professionals and caregivers. Current educational models disproportionately reflect services as a direct practice model. What we have learned from this project is that student-therapists are capable of learning to function in both consultative and direct service roles as new graduates. This is done effectively when new graduates develop the skills of knowing how to define the role of occupational therapy within a community setting, knowing their own limitations, using available resources and seeking regular supervision for validation of their clinical reasoning. Finally, at a time when community practice is expanding, it is important to provide such fieldwork experiences for students so they will be able to meet the growing demand for new positions in the community.

REFERENCES

Beer, D. & Helfrich, C. (1996). Chicago Homeless Head Start Demonstration Project Evaluation, University of Illinois at Chicago, Department of Occupational Therapy.

Bruffee, K.A. (1987). The art of collaborative learning. *Change*, 19, 2, 42-47.

Bruffee, K.A. (1995). Sharing our toys: Cooperative learning versus collaborative learning. *Change*, 27, 1, 12-18.

Curtin, C. & Baron, K.B. (1990). *The children's self assessment of occupational functioning.* Chicago, IL: Model of Human Occupation Clearinghouse, Department of Occupational Therapy, University of Illinois at Chicago.

Herge, E.A. & Milbourne, S.A. (1999). Self-directed learning: A model for occupational therapy fieldwork. In P.A. Crist (Ed.), *Innovations in occupational therapy education* (pp. 135-146). Bethesda, MD: American Occupational Therapy Association.

Kielhofner, G. (1992). *Conceptual foundations of occupational therapy* (2nd ed.). Philadelphia: F.A. Davis Company.

Knowles, M. & Associates (1984). *Andragogy in action.* San Francisco: Jossey-Bass.

Logan, B. & Dawkins, C. (1986). *Family-centered nursing in the community.* Menlo Park, CA: Addison-Wesley Publishing Co.

Mardell-Czudnowski, C. & Goldenberg, D.S. (1990). *Developmental Indicators for the Assessment of Learning-Revised (DIAL-R).* Circle Pines, MN: American Guidance Services.

Martens, K. (1981). Self-directed learning: An option for nursing education. *Nursing Outlook*, 29, 472-477.

Miller, L.J. (1993). *First step: Screening test for evaluating preschoolers.* San Antonio, TX: The Psychological Corporation Harcourt Brace Jovanovich, Inc.

Minkler, M. (Ed.). (1997). *Community organizing and community building for Health.* New Brunswick, NJ: Rutgers University Press.

Shugars, D.A., O'Neil, E.H., & Bader, J.D. (Eds.) (1991). *Healthy America: Practitioners for 2005, an agenda for action for U.S. health professional schools.* Durham, NC: The Pew Health Professions Commission.

Soto, M.A., Berhrens, R., & Rosemont, C. (Eds.) (1990). *Healthy people 2000.* Washington, DC: National Academy Press.

Townsend, S., Carey, P., Hollins, N., Helfrich, C., Blondis, M., Hoffman, A., Collins, L., & Blackwell, A. (2000). *The occupational therapy psychosocial assessment of learning.* Chicago, IL: Model of Human Occupation Clearinghouse, Department of Occupational Therapy, University of Illinois at Chicago.

Tresolini, C.P. & Shugars, D.A. (1994). An integrated health care model in medical education: Interviews with faculty and administration. *Academic Medicines*, 69, 3, 231-236.

Walens, D. (1997). *Professional behavior self-assessment.* University of Illinois at Chicago, Department of Occupational Therapy.

Walens, D., Wittman, P., Dickie, V., Kannenberg, K.R., Tomlinson, J.L., & Raynor,

O.U. (1998). Current and future education and practice: Issues for occupational therapy practitioners in mental health settings. *Occupational Therapy in Mental Health*. 14,1/2, 107-118. New York: The Haworth Press, Inc.

Walter, C.L. (1997). Community built practice: A conceptual framework. In M. Minkler (Ed.), *Community organizing and community building for health*. New Brunswick, NJ: Rutgers University Press.

Wiley, K. (1983). Effects of a self-directed learning project and preferences for structure on self directed learning readiness. *Nursing Research*, 32, 3, 181-185.

Occupational Therapy
and Victim Advocacy:
Making the Connection

Mark Koch, OTR/L

SUMMARY. This article provides an orientation to increase the profession's awareness of occupational therapy's role in victim advocacy, an emerging area of community-based practice. Analysis and comparison of OT's core assumptions and values with general principles of victim advocacy and empowerment demonstrate striking similarities: Each acknowledges holism and a profound connection between the individual and society, as well as their ability to interact and influence each other. In addition, the cultures of OT and victim advocacy both value the dignity and worth of persons, self-determination, freedom and autonomy, latent capacity, human uniqueness and subjectivity, and active and mutual cooperation in restoration or recovery. The compatibility of OT and victim advocacy is further demonstrated in the context of one therapist's work with survivors of domestic and sexual violence. *[Article copies available for a fee from The Haworth Document Delivery Service: 1-800-342-9678. E-mail address: <getinfo@haworthpressinc.com> Website: <http://www.HaworthPress.com> © 2001 by The Haworth Press, Inc. All rights reserved.]*

KEYWORDS. Domestic violence, sexual violence, victim advocacy, community-based practice

Mark Koch is Program Director, Coalition Against Rape and Domestic Violence, P.O. Box 786, Fulton, MO 65251.

[Haworth co-indexing entry note]: "Occupational Therapy and Victim Advocacy: Making the Connection." Koch, Mark. Co-published simultaneously in *Occupational Therapy in Mental Health* (The Haworth Press, Inc.) Vol. 16, No. 3/4, 2001, pp. 97-110; and: *Domestic Abuse Across the Lifespan: The Role of Occupational Therapy* (ed: Christine A. Helfrich) The Haworth Press, Inc., 2001, pp. 97-110. Single or multiple copies of this article are available for a fee from The Haworth Document Delivery Service [1-800-342-9678, 9:00 a.m. - 5:00 p.m. (EST). E-mail address: getinfo@haworthpressinc.com].

In order to be a true advocate, it is critical to change beliefs and accept truths about domestic violence. (Missouri Coalition Against Domestic Violence, 1998, p. 9)

Over the last quarter of the twentieth century, domestic and sexual violence emerged as major threats to the health and well-being of women and children in the United States (U.S. Department of Justice, 1998). For many survivors, the reality of being trapped by repeated assaults and coercion is equivalent to living in a war zone. Consequently, the negative impact of experiencing familial abuse can be devastating for children. Research has even demonstrated a generational link between childhood exposure to violence in the home and mental health problems later in life (Henning, Leitenberg, Coffey, Turner, & Bennett, 1996).

Although the prevalence and severity of domestic and sexual abuse have been well-documented, contemporary society has largely failed to address these issues. Recent increases in public and private spending have led to improvements in overall awareness and initial response; however, many cultural institutions (i.e., education, health care, social services, etc.) remain ignorant and unresponsive to the reality of those experiencing intimate violence and coercion. This lack of information and scarcity of adequate training reinforce the isolation that perpetuates victimization. Failure to break the cycle of violence imposes an enormous cost to society and individuals. While the annual medical expense of violent crimes is estimated in the billions (Miller, Cohen, & Rossman, 1993), the loss of human potential is immeasurable.

In the absence of uniform, public policies and educational initiatives that focus on a comprehensive response to victims, the battered women's, or advocacy, movement has relied considerably on the individual efforts of local grassroots coalitions to raise awareness and coordinate victim service. This has resulted in an uneven distribution of information and support. While advocates and their allies have argued that the most effective interventions involve a coordinated community response, some health care practitioners, including occupational therapists, have not taken an active role in collaborations. For many, it seems as if it has been easier to ignore, than to accept, that intimate abuse is a fundamental health care imperative. The Medical Power and Control Wheel (Figure 1) illustrates how such ignorance creates an ineffective health care response that re-victimizes battered women.

FIGURE 1. The Medical Power & Control Wheel

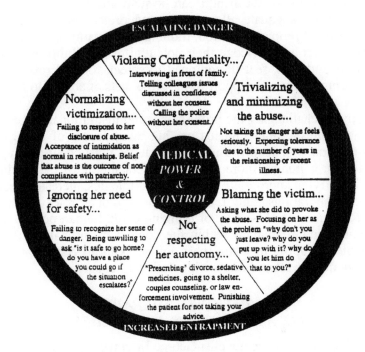

"The Medical Power & Control Wheel"*
Developed by the
Domestic Violence Project, Inc.
3556 7th Ave., Kenosha, WI 53140
(414) 656-3500

*Modeled after the "Power & Control and Equality Wheels" developed by the Domestic Abuse Intervention Project, 206 West 4th St., Duluth, MN 55806 (218) 722-4134

Today most major health care disciplines have adopted uniform guidelines and standards of practice for working with battered women (Stark & Flitcraft, 1996), yet professional literature regarding the occupational therapist's role in addressing victims' needs is grossly deficient. Accordingly, occupational therapists report that relatively few OT programs give sufficient attention to the dynamics of domestic and sexual violence and their impact on occupational performance (Johnston, Adams, & Helfrich, 2001). It should not be surprising that occupational therapists' (OTs) reluctance to address violence against women is a mirror of the health care system and society's broader failure to afford adequate attention to, and protection for, battered women. Without proper education, training, or empathy, occupational therapists do not acknowledge their potential responsibility in assisting victims and thus, feel ill-equipped to screen for and respond to those needing safety and support from further acts of abuse (Johnston, Adams, & Helfrich, 2001).

Effectively challenging the professional and institutional ignorance regarding domestic abuse means peeling away layers of disregard, misinformation, and apathy. Therefore, changes must occur on a variety of levels: gaining a more accurate understanding of the victim's reality, identifying appropriate intervention strategies, increasing community collaborations, and redefining professional roles (Wilson, 1997). Reexamining OTs' way of thinking about human occupation, dysfunction, and adaptation within the context of intimate violence will enable therapists to adapt their unique skills to coordinate and implement quality interventions with victims of abuse.

OCCUPATIONAL THERAPY: CORE ASSUMPTIONS AND VALUES

Over a century ago, the novelist George Eliot wrote, "It is never too late to be what you might have been" (Chaffee, 1998). Indeed, the culture of occupational therapy has always focused on transforming people's lives through being, doing, and ultimately becoming (Wilcock, 1999). Nearly eighty years ago, Adolph Meyer (1922) asserted the necessity of occupation in daily life. Two decades later, occupational therapists were applying this notion to the care and rehabilitation of casualties from two world wars. As moral treatment gave way to the mechanistic paradigm, the result was a crisis of confusion within the profession. Since then, OT has attempted to reclaim its foundation in occupation while embracing a more holistic and open framework to include the mind, body, and environment. Kielhofner (1992, pp. 48-49) refers to this "emerging paradigm of occupational therapy" as a model which reflects the following three assumptions:

1. Human beings have an occupational nature.
2. Human beings may experience occupational dysfunction.
3. Occupation can be used as a therapeutic agent.

Furthermore, Kielhofner (1992, p. 76) describes the values which shape the profession's practice:

Occupational therapy's values affirm human dignity and worth and the right of persons to their own perspectives and to self-determination. These values also recognize the importance of building on an individual's capacities, however limited, by allowing participation in occupation as a means of achieving a more healthy state. These values also ensure the person's right to compassionate care as they struggle to attain or maintain a level of function.

From the beginning, it has been the consistent demonstration of these core assumptions and values which has enabled OT to provide unique solutions to the restoration of individuals and society; however, as a profession, OT has ignored the casualties of another war that has been fought by a silent majority for centuries. Certainly, the profession exists because "it has an implicit social contract to address the problems of those members of society who have limited capacity to perform in their everyday occupations" (Kielhofner, 1992, p. 3). Yet, for the victims and survivors of domestic and sexual violence who are finally gaining access to health care institutions, OT has not kept its promise to address the needs of the time. Thus, the profession seems stuck between the progress of recognizing social change and the transformation to a sensitive, appropriate, and collaborative response to victims and survivors of domestic and sexual violence. Further, OT needs to coordinate this response with other health care professionals and with victim advocates.

PRINCIPLES OF VICTIM ADVOCACY AND EMPOWERMENT

Bolstered by the feminist and anti-rape movements of the 60s and 70s, the battered women's movement arose from the need of a flood of victims who turned to the earliest advocacy services in the country for support (Jones, 1994). In the 1970s with the establishment of the first rape crisis hotline in Washington, D.C., and the first domestic violence shelter in St. Paul, Minnesota, victims of domestic and sexual violence were finally given an opportunity to share their stories. Advocates engaged in these initiatives challenged the popular belief that violence in the home was a "private matter of the family" and introduced the abuse of power and control in intimate relationships as a public concern. They argued that abuse exists because of gender inequities and a history of oppression which subjugated women in society (Stalans & Lurigio, 1995).

By the mid 1970s, political leaders could no longer ignore the plight of abused women, and state governments began passing adult abuse protection laws, providing civil protection remedies (i.e., restraining or protective orders) for victims of intimate violence. In 1994, Congress passed the Violence Against Women Act (VAWA) to improve the safety of women nationwide. The VAWA not only increased penalties for some crimes against women but also provided for state grants to support law enforcement and educational programs aimed at reducing violent crimes against women. Despite these excellent strides, protection for survivors of domestic and sexual abuse is only as effective as the people who endorse or enforce such measures. As a result, the burden of safety often falls upon the victim herself as communities continue to struggle with challenging and changing the social acceptance of violence against women.

The core assumptions that underlie victim advocacy services for survivors of domestic abuse can be summarized into three areas:

1. The essential need for and right to safety,
2. The recognition that intimate violence and coercion pose unique challenges to the individual and society,
3. The value of empowerment in the restoration of survivors.

Advocates who empower and assist victims to well-being are concerned above all with the safety of the victim and her children. Safety is a basic human need (Maslow, 1954) and a fundamental right in any human relationship. Domestic and sexual violence are violations of that primary need for safety and security. Because a victim's greatest risk for harm occurs at the point in which she takes steps to end the abuse, every interaction and intervention must consider her safety and her assessment of the situation (Missouri Coalition Against Domestic Violence, 1999, p. 3).

In addition, domestic and sexual abuse are phenomena fraught with contradictions, working against the presupposition of mutuality and equality in a committed relationship. Explaining the victim's experience, Bard and Sangrey (1986, pp. 8-9) write that

> People can adjust to reality when they know what to expect. Experiences that meet our expectations are easier to handle, even if they are difficult and painful. But whenever experience fails to meet expectations, a person's ability to cope is compromised.

This description underscores the profound difficulties that many women face in accepting the dynamics of abuse within a relationship where love and intimacy coexist with power and control. Furthermore, it illustrates the enormous challenge facing communities struggling to accept that intimate violence simply exists. Recognition of this challenge can assist advocates in their efforts to validate and restore the survivor in her community which often blames the victim or ignores her situation.

Furthermore, advocacy services for battered women have always been founded on basic principles of empowerment. In Webster's Ninth New Collegiate Dictionary (1986), empowerment is defined as "investing with power or the right to act." For the purposes of advocacy, to empower is to assist, facilitate, help, support, and ultimately restore the individual. "Empowerment affords a battered woman the opportunity to see herself as a strong survivor who can participate actively in securing a safe and independent life" (Missouri Coalition Against Domestic Violence, 1999, p. 27). Developed by the Domestic Violence Project, Inc. in Kenosha, Wisconsin, The Empowerment Wheel highlights six ways in which advocates and others, who work with victims of domestic and sexual violence, can help to restore the individual to well-being. (See Figure 2.)

The philosophical underpinnings of empowerment will be further discussed in the next section as comparisons are drawn between the core assumptions and values of OT and victim advocacy.

MAKING THE CONNECTION

Domestic and sexual abuse should not be viewed as social ills to be eradicated or ignored. Through the skillful eyes of an OT, they might be perceived as Christiansen (1999) asserts, as "assaults of meaning,

FIGURE 2. The Empowerment Wheel

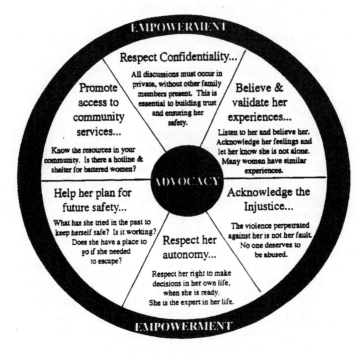

"The Advocacy Wheel"*
Developed by the
Domestic Violence Project, Inc.
3556 7th Ave., Kenosha, WI 53140
(414) 656-3500

*Modeled after the "Power & Control and Equality Wheels" developed by the Domestic Abuse Intervention Project, 206 West 4th St., Duluth, MN 55806 (218) 722-4134

phenomena that cause individuals to lose their sense of purpose and meaning in life." As one survivor of domestic violence explained:

> You cannot emerge a whole human being when you escape someone who constantly beats and berates you physically, emotionally, and spiritually. Until that searing of the soul has been attended to . . . There is something which happens to the psyche. The wholeness of the individual must be looked at. They must begin to understand what has happened to them and why. (Raphael & Tolman, 1997, p. 8)

This statement reflects many fundamental OT beliefs: a holistic understanding of identity and well-being, an appreciation of the multi-faceted nature of occupational performance, dysfunction, and adaptation, and acknowledgment of the inextricable link between the individual and the environment.

Further synthesis of victim advocacy with OT core assumptions and values reveals even more similarities. Themes that recognize the dignity and worth of individuals, validate the victim's experience, respect the right to autonomy, and promote active participation in restoration and recovery underlie empowerment. These same values guide OT practice, allowing the therapist to view the survivor's level of function as a result of adaptations rather than pathologies. Although both cultures acknowledge the assumption of safety for active participation in occupations, OT has been far less apt to practice this belief with battered women because the profession has largely ignored the victim's reality.

The work of an OT in a victim advocacy setting involves offering safety, support and resources to someone seeking refuge from violence and intimidation. Upon initial contact, the OT or advocate will assess the victim's risk for harm and begin gathering information to assist her in organizing a plan of action. This helps her take steps to regain control of her physical, emotional, social, financial, educational, and spiritual well-being. Because the level of involvement must be dictated by the particular needs of the individual seeking assistance, advocacy services will vary accordingly. While the OT may only need to inform some women about available community resources (i.e., housing, food, financial assistance, counseling and support, etc.), intervention may also include encouraging and facilitating participation in occupations once denied the victim. For example, with concurrent safety planning, the therapist can help the survivor find and secure employment after years of being denied the opportunity to work. Participation in employment is often restricted by the abusive partner who views this activity as a threat to his control. Overall, the challenge is not simply working with the victim of domestic violence, but working with *this* particular victim of abuse and her individual needs.

OT becomes a crucial part of victim advocacy when therapists provide safe environments that empower people to explore their potential and achieve success in daily tasks that are essential to well-being. OT's unique perspective on role acquisition and identity can enhance the survivor's understanding of her situation and motivation to engage in meaningful activities. Participation in occupations are opportunities to express the self and to create an identity (Christiansen, 1999). When applied to the victim's reality, these activities are vital to the restoration of someone whose identity has been compromised or lost as a result of previous abuse. Within the frameworks of OT and victim advocacy, the therapist may validate a new identity or empower the victim to recover a role previously denied her. Ultimately, this work not only assists the individual but also restores her connection with the community.

THE ROLE OF AN OCCUPATIONAL THERAPIST WITHIN A COMMUNITY-BASED ADVOCACY PROGRAM

Over the last three years, I have worked in various aspects of victim advocacy service delivery. From volunteer board member to Victim Advocate to Program Director, each role has given me opportunities to apply my OT skills in order to enhance advocacy services in a rural community. For instance, utilization of activity analysis has enabled me to reduce the complex task of organizing and implementing an advocacy program into its components. This has facilitated my ability to assess the community's needs, author grant proposals, organize victim services, develop collaborations with community service providers (i.e., law enforcement, civil and criminal justice personnel, social service workers, etc.), and measure program efficacy.

As the characteristics of a community shape organizational goals, the needs and resources of individual battered women direct the level of service provision by OT. Some survivors only need the therapist to serve as a consultant, linking them with community resources they have been isolated from in the past. Others may benefit from more intensive case management services in which, after gaining relevant background information, the OT develops an individualized goal or action plan. Each situation requires that the therapist or advocate make a comprehensive initial assessment of the victim's safety, measuring her risk of harm with available resources and support. This can be especially challenging when the victim herself is in a state of crisis (i.e., physical, emotional, spiritual, etc.) or when the victim has a mental illness, developmental delay, physical disability, or other special need. Nevertheless, "All women should be screened for domestic violence, because it is too common and too serious a problem to remain unidentified" (American Physical Therapy Association, 1997, p. 9). Helfrich and Aviles (2001), provide a useful framework for assessing the role of OT. Their paper also provides examples of intervention at various levels.

Baum and Law (1998, p. 8) suggest that "we must initiate efforts to work with others in the community in order to integrate a range of services that promote, protect, and improve the health of the public." Regardless of my professional role, I have gained a heightened appreciation of OT's potential to offer significant and unique contributions in the area of victim services.

CONCLUSION

As a profession and as individuals, we must prepare ourselves for this truth: Domestic and sexual violence is a reality for countless individuals who may receive OT services within a health care setting as well as community-based practice. First and foremost, therapists must educate themselves about the cycle of abuse, its effects on occupation and identity, and how to safely empower survivors. Information gives all of us strength and empathy (Robin Warshaw, 1994, p. xxvi). Some therapists already have and others are willing to receive it. The rest we still need to worry about, but the rest are within our power to change. That potential to be agents of change in the lives of others and our communities must be OT's greatest motivation to offer its unique understanding and expertise in building a nonviolent future for everyone. OT must assist in constructing a sensitive, appropriate, and coordinated response that asks each survivor what she needs to repair the harm of abuse.

Organizations, Agencies, and Coalitions

Center for the Prevention of Sexual and Domestic Violence
936 N. 34th Street, Suite 200
Seattle, WA 98103
Telephone: (206) 634-1903
www.cpsdv.org

Domestic Violence Initiative/Women With Disabilities
Post Office Box 300535
Denver, CO 80203
Telephone: (303) 839-5510
www.vs2000.org

National Coalition Against Domestic Violence (NCADV)
P. O. Box 18749
Denver, CO 80218-0749
Telephone: (303) 839-1852
www.ncadv.org

National Domestic Violence Hotline
P. O. Box 16180
Austin, TX 78716
Telephone: (800) 799-7233

Office for Victims of Crime Resource Center (OVCRC)
P. O. Box 6000
Rockville, MD 20849-6000
Telephone: (800) 627-6872
www.ncjrs.com

Recommended Reading

Davies, Jill. (1998). *Safety Planning with Battered Women: Complex Lives/Difficult Choices.* Thousand Oaks, CA: Sage Publications.
Evans, Patricia. (1987). *The Verbally Abusive Relationship.* Seattle: The Seal Press.
Fortune, Marie. (1987). *Keeping the Faith.* New York: Harper & Row.
Jones, Ann. (1995). *Next Time She'll Be Dead.* New York: Fawcett Columbine.
Pence, Ellen. (1987). *In Our Best Interest: A Process for Personal and Social Change.* Duluth, MN: Minnesota Program Development, Inc.
Roberts, Albert R. (Ed.) (1996). *Helping Battered Women.* New York: Oxford University Press.
Weiss, Elaine. (2000). *Surviving Domestic Violence: Voices of Women Who Broke Free.* Salt Lake City, UT: Agreka Books.

REFERENCES

American Physical Therapy Association. (1997). *Guidelines for recognizing and providing care for victims of domestic violence*. Alexandria, VA: American Physical Therapy Association.

Bard, M., & Sangrey, D. (1986). *The crime victim's book*. Secaucus, NJ: Citadel Press.

Baum, C., & Law, M. (1998). Community health: A responsibility, an opportunity, and a fit for occupational therapy. *The American Journal of Occupational Therapy, 52 (1)*, 7-10.

Chaffee, J. (1998). *The thinker's way: 8 steps to a richer life*. Boston: Little Brown & Company.

Christiansen, C.H. (1999). Defining lives: Occupation as identity: An essay on competence, coherence, and the creation of meaning. 1999 Eleanor Clark Slagle Lecture. *The American Journal of Occupational Therapy, 53*, 547-558.

Helfrich, C. & Aviles, A. (2001). OT's role with victims of domestic violence: Assessment and intervention. *Occupational Therapy in Mental Health, 16, 3/4* 53-70.

Henning, K., Leitenberg, H., Coffey, P., Turner, T., & Bennett, R.T. (1996). Long-term psychological and social impact of witnessing physical conflicts between parents. *Journal of Interpersonal Violence, 11*, 35-51.

Johnston, J.L., Adams, R., & Helfrich, C. (2001). Knowledge and attitudes of occupational therapy practitioners regarding wife abuse. *Occupational Therapy in Mental Health, 16, 3/4* 35-52.

Jones, A. (1995). *Next time she'll be dead*. New York: Fawcett Columbine.

Kielhofner, G. (1992). *Conceptual foundations of occupational therapy*. Philadelphia: F.A. Davis Company.

Maslow, A. (1954). *Motivation and personality*. New York: Harper.

Meyer, A. (1922). The philosophy of occupation therapy. *Archives of Occupational Therapy, 1*, 1-10.

Miller, T.R., Cohen, M.A., & Rossman, S.B. (1993). Victim costs of violent crime resulting injuries. *Health Affairs, 12*, 186-197.

Mish, F.C. et al. (Eds.) (1986). *Webster's ninth new collegiate dictionary*. Springfield, MA: Merriam-Webster Inc.

Missouri Coalition Against Domestic Violence. (1998). *The start-up manual: A workbook for new domestic violence service providers* (2nd ed.). Jefferson City, MO: Missouri Coalition Against Domestic Violence.

Missouri Coalition Against Domestic Violence. (1999). *The nature and dynamics of domestic violence: A curriculum for the Missouri department of social services*. Jefferson City, MO: Missouri Coalition Against Domestic Violence.

Raphael, J., & Tolman, R.M. (1997). *Trapped by poverty, trapped by abuse: New evidence documenting the relationship between domestic violence and welfare*. Chicago: Taylor Institute.

Stalans, L.J., & Lurigio, A.J. (1995). Two perspectives on domestic violence. In L. Gerdes (Ed.), *Battered women* (pp. 15-22). San Diego, CA: Greenhaven Press, Inc.

Stark, E., & Flitcraft, A. (1996). *Women at risk: Domestic violence and women's health*. Thousand Oaks, CA: Sage Publications.

U.S. Department of Justice, Bureau of Justice Statistics. (1998). *Violence by intimates: Analysis of data on crimes by current or former spouses, boyfriends, and girlfriends.*

Warshaw, R. (1994). *I never called it rape: The ms. report on recognizing, fighting, and surviving date and acquaintance rape.* New York: Harperperennial Library.

Wilcock, A.A. (1999). Reflections on doing, being, and becoming . . . (Abstract). *Canadian Journal of Occupational Therapy, 65,* 248.

Wilson, K.J. (1997). *When violence begins at home: A comprehensive guide to understanding and ending domestic abuse.* Alameda, CA: Hunter House Publishers.

PART III

Shaken Baby Syndrome: Assessment and Treatment in Occupational Therapy

Shannon LaEace MacDonald, OTR/L
Christine A. Helfrich, PhD, OTR/L

SUMMARY. Shaken Baby Syndrome is a serious form of child abuse, involving infants under the age of six months. Deliberately shaking an infant is often associated with frustration or anger, particularly when an infant will not stop crying. The shaking results in numerous initial and long-term consequences for the developing infant. In its most severe form Shaken Baby Syndrome results in the death of the infant. A case study detailing the clinical findings and treatment of a six-month-old infant with Shaken Baby Syndrome who received inpatient occupa-

Shannon LaEace MacDonald is Staff Therapist, The Rehabilitation Institute of Chicago, 345 East Superior, Chicago IL 60611 (E-mail: *SMACDONALD@rehabchicago.org*).

Christine A. Helfrich is Assistant Professor, Department of Occupational Therapy, University of Illinois at Chicago, 1919 W. Taylor Street (M/C 811), Chicago, IL 60612 (E-mail: *Helfrich@uic.edu*).

This article was completed in partial fulfillment of a Masters Degree in Occupational Therapy from the University of Illinois at Chicago. The authors would like to thank Kate Miller, OTR/L, for her support, mentoring and feedback in relation to this article.

[Haworth co-indexing entry note]: "Shaken Baby Syndrome: Assessment and Treatment in Occupational Therapy." MacDonald, Shannon LaEace, and Christine A. Helfrich. Co-published simultaneously in *Occupational Therapy in Mental Health* (The Haworth Press, Inc.) Vol. 16, No. 3/4, 2001, pp. 111-125; and: *Domestic Abuse Across the Lifespan: The Role of Occupational Therapy* (ed: Christine A. Helfrich) The Haworth Press, Inc., 2001, pp. 111-125. Single or multiple copies of this article are available for a fee from The Haworth Document Delivery Service [1-800-342-9678, 9:00 a.m. - 5:00 p.m. (EST). E-mail address: getinfo@haworthpressinc.com].

111

tional therapy services is presented. *[Article copies available for a fee from The Haworth Document Delivery Service: 1-800-342-9678. E-mail address: <getinfo@haworthpressinc.com> Website: <http://www.HaworthPress.com> © 2001 by The Haworth Press, Inc. All rights reserved.]*

KEYWORDS. Shaken baby syndrome, child abuse, occupational therapy

INTRODUCTION

In the field of occupational therapy it is almost certain a therapist will provide intervention for someone who is a victim of violence. Unfortunately, violence is all too common with youth and children. School aged children have even become victims in their own schools by other classmates. Yet, far more disturbing than violence in the schools is violence in the home. The home is supposed to be a safe and loving environment that facilitates growth and development. However, the home is not immune to violence. Each year 160,000 children suffer severe or life-threatening injuries and 1-2,000 children die as a result of abuse (Bethea, 1999). Children under one year of age make up 40% of child abuse victims and homicide is the leading cause of injury-related deaths in this age group (Bethea, 1999; Committee on Child Abuse and Neglect, 1993-1994). Injuries that result in the death of an infant are rarely unintentional unless there is an obvious explanation, such as a motor vehicle crash. Billmire and Meyers (1985) determined that when uncomplicated skull fractures were excluded, 95% of serious intracranial injuries and 64% of all head injuries in infants were due to child abuse.

RISK FACTORS FOR CHILD ABUSE

Prior to 1986, when Bergman and colleagues studied severe abusive injuries, mothers were thought to be the most common perpetrators of child abuse. This study concluded that males (fathers and mothers' boyfriends) were the most common perpetrators of severe child abuse cases resulting in permanent injury or even death (Bergman, Larsen & Mueller, 1986). Starling, Holden and Jenny (1995) further supported Bergman and colleagues' findings. Men were found to be 2.2 times more likely to commit crimes of abuse. These data imply that men are at a greater risk to abuse infants. After males, babysitters were the most likely perpetrators of abuse, a previously unrecognized group of possible abusers (Starling et al., 1995). Mothers were found to be the least frequent abusers among all identified perpetrators.

According to the 1990 census report, 60% of mothers of preschoolers work outside of the home (Starling et al., 1995). This suggests that many mothers are not the primary caretakers of their children. The responsibility of child care may be left to males and/or babysitters. Since it was previously believed that mothers were the abusers and the primary caregivers, it is important to redirect prevention efforts to target males and babysitters who may actually be the primary caregiver and may be a greater risk for becoming abusers.

There are a number of risk factors which compound a person's tendency to become a child abuser or become a victim of child abuse (Bethea, 1999). (See Table 1.)

SHAKEN BABY SYNDROME

The term Shaken Baby Syndrome has evolved since initially coined "whiplash shaken baby syndrome" in 1972, by John Caffey, a pediatric radiologist, to describe a number of clinical findings in infants (Committee on Child Abuse and Neglect, 1993-1994). These findings included retinal hemorrhages, subdural and/or subarachnoid hemorrhages, with little or no evidence of external cranial trauma (Duhaime, Christian, Rorke & Zimmerman, 1998; Krous & Byard, 1999; Starling et al., 1995). A year earlier it was concluded that the whiplash forces caused subdural hematomas by tearing the cortical bridging veins (Committee on Child Abuse and Neglect, 1993-1994). While a number of supporters have expanded on Caffey's findings, he also met some challengers. Duhaime et al. (1998) questioned whether or not shaking alone could cause these clinical findings. They found that rather than the actual shaking, the force of rapid deceleration of a shaken head hitting any surface, such as a bed or pillow, might be the basis for most of these serious injuries (Duhaime et al., 1998).

Shaken Baby Syndrome is considered a serious form of child maltreatment involving children younger than six months of age (Becker, Liersch, Tautz, Schlueter & Andler, 1998). In order to be labeled Shaken Baby Syndrome the shaking must be of such a force that even

TABLE 1. Child Abuse Risk Factors

RISK ORIGIN	RISK FACTORS
COMMUNITY/SOCIETAL	1. High crime rate 2. Lack of or few social services 3. High poverty rate 4. High unemployment rate
PARENT-RELATED	1. Personal history of being abused 2. Teenage parents 3. Single parent 4. Emotional immaturity 5. Poor coping skills 6. Low self-esteem 7. Personal history of substance abuse 8. Known history of child abuse 9. Lack of social support 10. Domestic violence 11. Lack of parenting skills 12. History of depression 13. History of mental illness 14. Multiple young children 15. Unwanted pregnancy 16. Denial of pregnancy
CHILD-RELATED	1. Prematurity 2. Low birth weight 3. Handicapped

a lay person would recognize the act as dangerous. The shaking occurs repeatedly and rapidly and the child may or may not be thrown onto a couch or other surface, creating an impact. When an infant is shaken, the brain jerks back and forth in the skull, resulting in a coup and counter coup injury to the brain. Blood vessels in and around the brain are damaged and can begin to bleed into the brain causing further damage. In its most severe form, Shaken Baby Syndrome results in the death of the infant. In the mildest of cases it is overlooked and under-diagnosed appearing as if the infant is sleeping.

Risk Factors for Shaken Baby Syndrome

Deliberately shaking an infant is most often associated with frustration or anger, particularly when an infant will not stop crying. The combination of a crying baby and a frustrated caregiver can result in Shaken Baby Syndrome. A number of incidences have been identified as triggering events of Shaken Baby Syndrome. Triggering events can occur in isolation or there can be a combination of triggering events (Duhaime et al., 1998; Bethea, 1999). These triggering events include:

- An inadequately prepared parent
- A caregiver under stress
- Multiple births (i.e., twins)
- Having multiple children under eighteen months of age
- A child with a disability
- Teenage parents
- A caregiver with poor coping skills
- Substance abuse among the caregiver
- Economic strains and poverty
- Difficulty soothing or calming a crying infant

Implications of Shaken Baby Syndrome

The effects of shaking a baby can be devastating. If the shaking is enough to produce the clinical findings of Shaken Baby Syndrome, the infant will suffer initial consequences as well as long-term consequences. Shaken Baby Syndrome is recognized as one of the most frequent causes of traumatic mortality and morbidity in infants (Duhaime et al., 1996). Infants with this condition vary in presentation. The infant can have neurological complications which may present as seizures, difficulty breathing, limp arms and legs, excessive drooling, lethargy, or death. The long-term effects of shaking a baby may include seizure disorder, learning impairments, physical impairments, speech impairments, visual impairments, and hearing impairments. Each of these factors complicates treatment and intervention for the infant.

As previously stated, infants with a disability are at higher risk for abuse. Therefore, an infant with impairments due to Shaken Baby Syndrome is now at a greater risk for future abuse secondary to the disabling conditions that resulted from the initial brain damage. The outcome for infants who have this condition is not favorable. In 1996, Duhaime et al. closely investigated the long-term consequences of shaking an infant. Fourteen children were contacted at an average of nine years after injury. Of the fourteen children contacted, six were boys and eight were girls, with an average age of 6.4 months at the time of injury.

At the time of injury, the infants presented to the emergency room with varying conditions. Six of the children were lethargic or irritable, three children experienced seizures without being in a coma, and five presented in a coma either with or without seizures (Duhaime et al., 1996). Of the fourteen infants twelve had retinal hemorrhages. All of the infants' acute CT scans indicated subarachnoid and/or subdural blood in the brain. Seven of the infants were intubated in the acute phases for apnea, seizures, and/or unresponsiveness. All of the infants were provided standard treatment for a head injury, including monitoring in the intensive care unit.

Nine years later, during the follow-up study, one child who was in a persistent vegetative stage had died from respiratory complications. Six of the children remained severely impaired and vegetative, two were moderately impaired, and five were said to have a good outcome (Duhaime et al., 1996). Of those six children identified as having a severe impairment, three were legally blind, nonverbal, and wheelchair bound; one child was legally blind, mentally impaired, and had a seizure disorder; and two children had hemiparesis, severe learning impairments and behavioral problems. The two children who were identified as having moderate impairments experienced visual impairments, difficulties with cognition requiring special education; and one of the two children also had mild hemiparesis. The five children who were labeled as having a good outcome were attending regular schools; however, three out of the five were required to repeat a grade or to receive tutoring in order to supplement their typical school day. In addition to the necessity to repeat grades and be tutored, two of the children also had behavioral difficulties (Duhaime et al., 1996). These clinical findings suggest that a majority of infants who experience the Shaken Baby Syndrome will encounter long-term functional impairments.

CASE STUDY

Background Information

John (all names have been changed for anonymity) is a 6-month-old infant who presented for inpatient acute rehabilitation three weeks after an insult to his brain. Prior to this incident, it was reported that

John was developing normally. John is the first child to unmarried teenage parents, Kelly, 16-years-old, and Paul, 17-years-old. It is not known whether or not the pregnancy was desired. Kelly and Paul lived with their own parents prior to the birth of John and moved in together after his birth. Both John and Kelly worked full-time on opposite shifts and did not use outside child care. Because they were working full-time on opposite shifts, all parenting was performed independently of each other. Each parent was alone with John throughout the day. Kelly and Paul found that they had no time alone together and no respite from child care and full-time employment.

One evening, after returning home from work, Kelly found John in his crib asleep. After a few hours she attempted to wake him for his feeding. John was difficult to arouse and appeared tired and was unable to nurse; however, John was not crying. The next morning when Kelly woke up she found it strange that John did not wake up during the night. When she attempted to nurse him, he was uninterested and appeared very limp. Kelly called the doctor who requested Kelly take the baby to the emergency room.

Initial Examination

At the emergency room the physicians examined John. Both parents were separately asked questions regarding events of the evening. Kelly was away from the home at work and reported that John appeared normal when she left the home for work that evening. Paul reported that John was crying a great deal during the evening. After repeated attempts to console him with walking, changing his diaper, cuddling, and a bottle, John continued to cry. Paul reports feeling helpless and states " I started to toss him in the air to see if that would make him laugh or at least stop him from crying. It worked because John stopped crying and after a few minutes he closed his eyes and went to sleep in his crib." Paul's statement led the staff to suspect Shaken Baby Syndrome and that John may have brain damage.

A physician's initial examination revealed a bulging anterior fontanel. A CT scan revealed a previous blunt insult to the head, subarchoid hemorrhaging, and various lesions in the brain. X-ray results indicated previous fractured ribs, which suggested possible previous abuse.

Reporting Child Abuse

Since child abuse was suspected in this incident, it was mandatory to notify the Department of Children and Family Services (DCFS) within 24 hours. DCFS was notified and intervention was provided immediately during the acute medical stay. DCFS began by taking a family history and investigating events surrounding the situation that led to the injury which has been identified as questionable abuse. DCFS assisted in determining a legal guardian for the infant and served as an advocate for the child insuring that decisions were made in John's best interest. In John's case, it was difficult to determine a legal guardian, as neither Kelly's nor Paul's parents would accept the responsibility of becoming a legal guardian. Ultimately, DCFS and the courts determined that Kelly's aunt would be the temporary legal guardian of John. This decision was made before John began his inpatient rehabilitation.

The court ruled that all visits by Kelly and/or Paul required supervision. Kelly's aunt or any member of the health care team could provide supervision during visitation. Under no circumstances were Kelly and/or Paul allowed to be alone with John in his hospital room. The rehabilitation team was also informed that the infant was not allowed off the unit. John's crib was placed in front of the nurse's station to allow for close monitoring of visitations, since the pediatric unit is unlocked. John remained on the inpatient rehabilitation unit for 21 days.

Occupational Therapy Intervention

Treating an infant with Shaken Baby Syndrome can be extremely challenging for an occupational therapist. Each infant varies in presenting functional deficits and family situations. While an inpatient, John received skilled occupational therapy, physical therapy, and speech therapy. All disciplines provided individual services daily for at least one hour, totaling three hours of therapy a day. Inpatient therapy services were an aggressive attempt to promote and facilitate normal motor development and remediate functional deficits, which occurred as a result of the brain damage. During the initial occupational therapy evaluation it was determined that John's development varied significantly from what would be typical of a child his age (Table 2).

Initially, John was an extremely challenging infant to treat. It was

TABLE 2. John's Development

Developmental Motor Control	Typical Development at 6 Months	John at 6 Months
Head Control	Fully developed.	Absent.
Vision	Infant visually tracks objects.	Left eye inwardly rotated; unable to visually track an object.
Auditory	Auditory interests influence head turning and transitional movements.	Absent startle reflex when presented with loud auditory stimuli.
Oral Motor	Able to take a bottle, or breast feed, may comfort self with a pacifier.	Impaired oral motor control; an insufficient suck for feeding.
Extremity Control	Dissociated movements of all extremities.	No voluntary movement of extremities.
Prone	Prone is a functional, mobile position. The infant can push up and weight shift on extended arms.	Unable to tolerate prone. Immediately cries when placed in the prone position.
Grasp	Initiates grasp and can crudely manipulate an object and bring it to the mouth.	Unable to maintain grasp on object when directly placed in infant's hand.
Sitting	Can sit independently without external support.	Requires total support while sitting.
Standing	When placed in standing can take full weight on lower extremities; begins to bounce by flexing and extending knees.	Extensor tone dominates lower extremities. Unable to be placed in a supported stance position secondary to inadequate head and neck control.
Reaching	Beginning to reach for toys when the trunk is supported.	No purposeful movements of upper extremities.
Transitions	Independent with transitions from supine to and from prone.	No active transitional movements. Does not tolerate passive rolling.
Range of Motion	All extremities easily move through full range of motion.	Resting position of both hands is with thumb adducted into palm; passive movement is mildly difficult secondary to increased tone in upper extremities.
Interaction with the Environment	Interacts with the environment appropriately.	No awareness of the environment.

evident that he had significant functional impairments. He appeared limp while being held, his left eye was inwardly deviated, and he had a nasal gastric tube for feedings.

During occupational therapy sessions it was essential to position an infant in proper developmental positions to promote age appropriate development. Initially, John was only comfortable while being held. When placed supine on the mat he immediately began assuming in an asymmetrical tonic neck reflex position (which indicates abnormal posturing known as the fencing position). In order to decrease this abnormal posturing John was positioned in sidelying. The sidelying position allows gravity to assist with bringing the arms to a midline position. While in a sidelying position, the occupational therapist passively brought John's hands to his mouth or a toy to encourage interaction between himself and the environment. In John's case, he was not able to visually attend to the environment, so hands to mouth was initiated by the therapist. When John's hands were brought to his mouth, he began to suck on his fingers.

John was placed in a supported sitting position during occupational therapy sessions, with the therapist providing external trunk support in order for John to maintain this position. John had limited head and trunk control. It was essential to assist John with a "supported sit" in order to allow for opportunities to strengthen neck extensors and facilitate head and neck control.

During the second week of occupational therapy John's muscle tone began to increase in both his upper and lower extremities. It became difficult to administer passive range of motion to John's upper extremities, especially his hands. John required bilateral resting hand splints to be worn throughout the day, two hours on and two hours off. The bilateral resting hand splints promoted proper positioning of the hands in order to maintain the arches and decrease spasticity. Ensuring that the splints were properly worn was a shared responsibility of all disciplines including occupational therapy. During the two hours while the resting hand splints were off, John wore soft neoprene thumb loop splints in order to properly position the thumb in extension and abduction.

As John's tolerance for various developmental positions increased, more challenging activities were introduced. John was able to tolerate a sidelying position for greater than twenty minutes on each side. He

was visually tracking to midline with his right eye. In order to facilitate John's tolerance of the prone position, which is necessary for
weightbearing through bilateral upper and lower extremities, John was
positioned prone over the occupational therapist's leg. This functional
position allowed weightbearing through bilateral lower extremities as
well as encouraged neck extension and upper extremities to midline.

During John's third week of therapy he took all meals by bottle.
Occasionally, his meal times were during occupational therapy sessions. While John was feeding, the occupational therapist would facilitate hands to midline in order for John to hold the bottle. Initially,
John required total assist to bring his hands to midline; however, at the
time of discharge he was independently bringing his hands to the
bottle during meal time. During meal times, it was important to facilitate proper positioning. Often he was positioned in a supported sit with
the occupational therapist on the mat, or he was seated in a chair that
provided proper positioning while seated.

Family Education and Training

Family teaching and training ideally should be an ongoing process
during an inpatient rehabilitation stay. However, in the case of many
infants with Shaken Baby Syndrome the legal guardian and/or discharge destination is unknown. Many times when an infant is placed in
a foster home, the infant will be discharged to the foster family without any training or education occurring.

In John's situation, Kelly's aunt had been identified as the legal
guardian so family training and education was an ongoing process.
Both Kelly and Paul were present along with the aunt for training and
education. The occupational therapist educated the family members on
typical development of an infant. John's family was educated on the
psychosocial and physical deficits that resulted from the brain damage. The occupational therapist validated the common feelings of
frustration that arise when caring for an infant, especially an inconsol-
able infant.

Impact of Inpatient Hospitalization on the Family and Infant

While John was an inpatient, Kelly and Paul visited at least three
times per week. During John's inpatient stay it was evident that bond-

ing between Kelly and John had been affected. Prior to this incident, John was being breast-fed by Kelly; now he was taking a bottle four times a day and numerous health care professionals were assisting with mealtimes. Also given the fact that all of Kelly's actions were monitored, her affection and actions towards John appeared extremely unnatural as though she was self-conscious. Kelly was having a difficult time adjusting to the changes in John. She stated that he appeared not to recognize her or even smile at her as he had done prior to this incident. The occupational therapist educated the family on the challenges that John now faced when socially interacting with others. These challenges were due to his visual, auditory, and motor impairments. All involved expressed their concerns over the lack of positive feedback they received while caring and interacting with John. Therefore, family teaching focused on the family's understanding of other positive feedback, besides smiling, that would suggest that John enjoyed their interaction (i.e., decreased fussiness and/or decreased muscle tone). Adjustment to a child with a disability can be difficult for any parent. This matter may have been compounded by the fact that Kelly and Paul were first-time parents. Now their child had numerous physical and social impairments.

DISCUSSION

The occupational therapist who works with an infant with the Shaken Baby Syndrome may experience a number of frustrations. It can be disturbing to realize that the incident could have been prevented. It is frustrating not to have a definitive discharge destination or date. And, it is extremely disturbing to encounter the suspected abuser during family training and education.

Encountering the effects of violence on an innocent victim such as a child may be difficult. There is a tremendous amount of frustration in knowing that the child's deficits could have been prevented; however, it is important that clinicians cast aside their anger and biases. It is helpful to remember that the opportunity to provide family teaching and training can be invaluable to the infant as well as the abuser. This training may be the only training the abuser ever receives in parenting or handling skills.

It can be frustrating when a discharge destination has not been determined for the infant. It is difficult when the team is only provided with a two-day notice that the infant will be placed in a foster home and the foster family will be unavailable for any training or education with the health care team. It is disturbing when a legal guardian has been identified and does not come to visit the child and is unable to attend scheduled family training and education sessions with the health care team.

The occupational therapist is expected to provide education and training to all caregivers, which may include suspected abusers. Providing education and training to child abusers can be difficult. Therapists may struggle with their anger towards the abuser as well as the supposed injustices in the child welfare system. There is an overall fear that this could happen again.

It is essential for the therapist to convey to caregivers that they are not taking home a healthy, typically developing child. Family members often appear to believe the infant is "cured" because he or she is being discharged from the hospital. The family, legal guardian or foster parent may not understand that the infant most likely will experience long-term deficits from the brain damage. This may be especially difficult to realize in infants, because to the lay person, the baby may not appear to do anything except eat or sleep.

CONCLUSIONS AND FURTHER RECOMMENDATIONS

The reality is that Shaken Baby Syndrome is preventable. Efforts to promote prevention should not only be directed at mothers but also toward men and babysitters. Often babysitters are required to participate in babysitting and infant CPR classes given by the American Red Cross prior to a babysitting job. Possibly new parents could benefit from this same type of instruction and training prior to childbirth. Increasing the amount of public service announcements regarding the dangers of shaking an infant could possibly be effective in prevention. Early detection by the primary care physician is crucial and should be routine during pregnancy and early infancy. Occupational therapists are well suited to provide education and intervention to the individual and the community. This will ultimately prevent child abuse. In order to successfully prevent child abuse the effort and intervention must occur at all levels.

The most important message to remember is that *it is never okay to shake a baby!*

National Information:

National Committee to Prevent Child Abuse
332 S. Michigan Ave., Suite 1600
Chicago, IL 60604-4357
Telephone: 312-663-3520
Fax: 312-939-8962
Website: *http://www.childabuse.org*

Support and Referral Service on Shaken Baby Syndrome
2955 Harrison Blvd., #102
Ogden, UT 84403
Telephone: 801-393-3366
Fax: 801-393-7019

REFERENCES

Becker, J.C., Liersch, R., Tautz, C., Schlueter, B., Andler, W. (1998). Shaken Baby Syndrome: Report on four pairs of twins. *Child Abuse and Neglect, 22 (9),* 931-937.

Bergman, A.B., Larsen, R.M., Mueller, B.A. (1986). Changing spectrum of serious child abuse. *Pediatrics, 77,* 113-116.

Bethea, L. (1999). Primary prevention of child abuse. *American Family Physician, 59 (6),* 1577-1585.

Billmire, M.E., Myers, P.A. (1995). Serious head injury in infants: Accident or abuse. *Pediatrics, 75,* 340-342.

Bly, L. (1994). *Motor skills acquisition in the first year.* Therapy Skill Builders, Harcourt Assessment Company, Tucson, AZ.

Duhaime, A., Christian, C., Moss, E., Seidl, F. (1996). Long-term outcomes in infants with the Shaking-Impact Syndrome. *Pediatric Neurosurgery, 24,* 292-298.

Duhaime, A., Christian, C., Rorke, L., Zummerman, R. (1998). Nonaccidental head injury in infants–"The Shaken-Baby Syndrome." *The New England Journal of Medicine, 338 (25),* 1822-1829.

Krous, H., Byard, R. (1999). Shaken Infant Syndrome: Selected controversies. *Pediatric and Developmental Pathology, 2,* 497-498.

Krugman, R., Lenherr, M., Betz, L., Fryer, G. (1986). The relationship between unemployment and physical abuse of children. *Child Abuse and Neglect (10)*, 415-418.

Lacey, M. (1998). Patterns of abuse in the home. *Home Care Provider, 3 (6)*, 319-323.

Starling, S.P., Holden, J.R., Jenny, C. (1995). Abusive head trauma. The relationship of perpetrators to their victims. *Pediatrics, 95 (2)*, 259-262.

The Committee on Child Abuse and Neglect. (1997). Shaken Baby Syndrome: Inflicted cerebral trauma. *Delaware Medical Journal, 69 (7)*, 365-70.

Child Witnesses of Domestic Violence: A Case Study Using the OT PAL

Jonathan Nave, OTS
Christine A. Helfrich, PhD, OTR/L
Ann Aviles, OTR/L

SUMMARY. Children who witness domestic violence experience a variety of negative effects. These include maladaptation in the areas of behavioral, emotional, social, cognitive, and physical functioning. The Occupational Therapy Psychosocial Assessment of Learning (OT PAL) is a tool that can be used to evaluate the psychosocial functioning of a student's performance in a classroom environment. Presented is the case study of a child witness of domestic violence and the use of the OT PAL in measuring the psychosocial aspects of his performance in a nontraditional classroom setting. *[Article copies available for a fee from The Haworth Document Delivery Service: 1-800-342-9678. E-mail address: <getinfo@haworthpressinc.com> Website: <http://www.HaworthPress.com> © 2001 by The Haworth Press, Inc. All rights reserved.]*

KEYWORDS. Domestic violence, pediatrics, assessment, occupational therapy

Jonathan Nave is an MSC student, Department of Occupational Therapy, University of Illinois at Chicago, 1919 W. Taylor Street (M/C 811), Chicago, IL 60612 (E-mail: *jnave1@uic.edu*).

Christine A. Helfrich is Assistant Professor, Department of Occupational Therapy, University of Illinois, Chicago, IL (E-mail: *Helfrich@uic.edu*).

Ann Aviles is Research Assistant, Department of Occupational Therapy, University of Illinois, Chicago, IL (E-mail: *aavile1@uic.edu*).

This article was completed in partial fulfillment of a Masters in Science Degree in Occupational Therapy from the University of Illinois at Chicago.

For questions pertaining to this article, please direct all correspondence to Dr. Christine Helfrich.

[Haworth co-indexing entry note]: "Child Witnesses of Domestic Violence: A Case Study Using the OT PAL." Nave, Jonathan, Christine A. Helfrich, and Ann Aviles. Co-published simultaneously in *Occupational Therapy in Mental Health* (The Haworth Press, Inc.) Vol. 16, No. 3/4, 2001, pp. 127-140; and: *Domestic Abuse Across the Lifespan: The Role of Occupational Therapy* (ed: Christine A. Helfrich) The Haworth Press, Inc., 2001, pp. 127-140. Single or multiple copies of this article are available for a fee from The Haworth Document Delivery Service [1-800-342-9678, 9:00 a.m. - 5:00 p.m. (EST). E-mail address: getinfo@haworthpressinc.com].

INTRODUCTION

It is estimated that at least 3.3 million children witness physical and verbal spousal abuse each year (Jaffe, Wolfe, & Wilson, 1990). Children who have witnessed domestic violence in the past have been labeled at risk and little more has been said about the effects of their experiences. Recently, more research has focused on the effects of children witnessing domestic violence. In a review of 29 articles researching the effects of children witnessing domestic violence, Kolbo, Blakely, and Engleman (1996) found that child witnesses are at risk for maladaptation in at least one area of behavioral, emotional, social, cognitive, or physical functioning. Similarly, Nelms (1994) stated that child witnesses of domestic violence may experience developmental delays in the areas of social, emotional, and cognitive development.

In an article on the psychological adjustments and competencies of child witnesses of domestic violence, children who witnessed verbal and physical violence between their parents displayed more behavior problems than a control group who did not witness violence in their home (Fantuzzo, DePaola, Lambert, Martino, Anderson, & Sutton, 1991). Children in families who became homeless to escape domestic violence also scored lower on scales of social competency and conflict reasoning (Fantuzzo et al., 1991). Additionally, young school-aged children in a battered women's shelter scored almost one standard deviation below the normative average in the area of self-concept (Hughs & Barad, 1983).

Thormaehlen and Bass-Feld (1994) in their article on the secondary victims of domestic violence stated that children may experience feelings of guilt, shame, lack of trust, poor self-esteem, helplessness, and hopelessness after witnessing domestic violence. In addition, they also explain that children's behavior may be affected. Children may exhibit difficulty controlling impulses and anger, and when they become frustrated, may resort to violence. Children may also exhibit difficulty in problem solving, and have an inability to communicate feelings in a healthy way. Additionally, the authors stated that child witnesses of domestic violence may fail to reach normal developmental milestones or even regress (e.g., bed-wetting after being toilet trained).

Occupational Therapy Assessments

The development of psychosocial skills is very important for children and has a strong impact on a child's ability to learn. Many of the components of social competence can be defined as psychosocial skills and are important to a child's functioning in a school setting. When a child is experiencing difficulty meeting expectations and roles within the classroom, it is very important for psychosocial skills to be considered as a possible cause of the difficulty. Components of social competence include motivation, self-esteem, personal causation and identification of one's roles and the expectations connected to these roles. All of these components contribute to the student's success in the classroom.

In the past, the occupational therapy profession lacked discipline specific assessments that address psychosocial aspects of being a student. There are numerous assessments that occupational therapists use to evaluate abilities in children that are related to development and function, but few of them address psychosocial issues. There are even fewer assessments used by occupational therapists that *focus* on psychosocial skills and none are designed specifically for assessing psychosocial skills in school-based settings. The *Occupational Therapy Psychosocial Assessment of Learning* (Townsend, Carey, Hollins, Helfrich, Blondis, Hoffman, Collins, & Blackwell, 2000) was developed to fill the need to measure the psychosocial aspects of a student's performance within the classroom as part of an occupational therapy evaluation.

The Occupational Therapy Psychosocial Assessment of Learning (OT PAL)

The OT PAL (Townsend et al., 2000) is an observational and descriptive assessment tool, targeted at students 6-12 years old who are having difficulty meeting the functional expectations and roles within the classroom. The OT PAL uses the Model of Human Occupation (Kielhofner, 1995) to address a student's volition (ability to make choices), habituation (roles and routines), and environmental fit within the classroom setting. The observational portion consists of 23 items divided into three major areas that include making choices, habits/routines, and roles that can be assessed in two 20-minute observations. These items are designed to facilitate the gathering of essential information regarding the student's behavior, the social expectations and physical environment of the classroom.

The OT PAL also includes a descriptive portion that consists of three semi-structured interviews for the teacher, the student, and the parent(s). The interviews are designed to have the teacher, student, and parent describe various psychosocial aspects of learning related to school and can be conducted as a written questionnaire and completed in approximately 15 minutes. Different perspectives gained through questions relating to the student's performance, behaviors, beliefs, and interests related to school are helpful in gaining a more holistic view of the child's performance.

CASE STUDY

Family History

Michael (all names have been changed for anonymity) is an 8-year-old biracial male. His father is Caucasian, and his mother is African-American. Michael is the third of four children in his family. He has an older brother and sister, and a younger brother. Michael's mother, Barbara, met his father in their senior year of high school and they married shortly after graduation; both parents were 18 years old. Both parents witnessed violence in their homes growing up, but neither parent had ever received counseling. Michael's mother explained that her abuse began gradually. Two months into the marriage, Michael's father began emotionally abusing her with threats of beatings whenever he had a bad day at work.

Michael's mother was 20 years old when she gave birth to him and at that time Michael's father was abusing her physically, emotionally, and sexually. Barbara expressed fear of leaving his father because he had threatened to kill her. She stated that until Michael was 7 years old he witnessed his father threaten and physically assault her regularly, but was never abused himself.

Michael was 7-1/2 years old when his mother left his father and took the children to a homeless shelter. She left after verbal and physical assault by the father. She explained that Michael's father did not let her have any friends and she had no family in the state so they became homeless. Michael and his family lived in a shelter for five days and were then referred to a transitional housing facility for women and their children who have become homeless after fleeing domestic violence. The transitional housing facility allows families to live there for up to two years while they work, go to school, or get their GED. Each family has their own apartment, and pays rent on a sliding scale according to income. The facility also has a day care program and a before and after school program for the children of the women who live there.

Michael

Michael and his family had been living in the transitional housing facility for six months when he began occupational therapy. Michael participated in the summer session of the Before and After School Program which ran daily from 8:00 a.m. to 6:30 p.m. The classroom was designed for students 6-12 years old. During the summer the program provides arts and crafts activities, field trips, and group activities to encourage the students to interact in a socially appropriate manner.

Over the summer the author worked with Michael in the classroom five days a week. Michael enjoyed playing Uno and one of his favorite games was fooseball (a table top soccer game). Michael also enjoyed making clay figures of Pokemon characters and was talented at building with Duplo blocks (a larger form of Legos). Michael also enjoyed kicking the ball around with adults, and going to the playground.

Michael was often aggressive and engaged in a physical altercation (punching in the face, kicking, etc.) with another member of the class almost daily. Michael would then consistently lie about his behavior, always saying that he was hit first. When asked to sit in the "time-out" chair as a consequence of his behavior, Michael would sometimes respond by having a tantrum. His tantrums involved loud dramatic crying and/or yelling. His tantrums usually included knocking over chairs, pushing adults, and/or throwing objects such as toys. Michael's tantrums usually lasted from 3-5 minutes, with one tantrum lasting just over 12 minutes. Michael had 3-5 minute tantrums at least twice a week.

When Michael seemed to be getting along and playing with the other students appropriately, he would suddenly punch one of them in the arm or pinch them on the back. Michael often laughed and smiled inappropriately such as when he or others in the class were being reprimanded or when others were hurt. If the other kids in the class were talking about something he did not know, such as a television show he had not seen, Michael used nonsensical words that the other children did not understand. Michael also exhibited some inappropriate sexual hand gestures about once a week.

Michael demonstrated cognitive difficulty as well. Michael's mother reported that his academic performance was poor, but passing. When Michael was involved in art making or craft activities he often would begin the activity by refusing to do it. With encouragement, he would participate but quit before finished, throwing down whatever materials he was using, saying he did not understand how to do it or that the activity was "too hard," or "stupid." Michael would sometimes call himself stupid if asked what was too hard for him to do.

DISCUSSION

Michael's treatment plan consisted of several recommendations for the classroom staff to implement in the classroom and addressed his need for further formal assessment of his fine and gross motor skills. The need for the first part of the plan, "development of a behavior modification program that is consistent and present oriented," was identified by Item I of Making Choices and through the analysis of the student-environmental fit. One way that this recommendation could be carried out is through the use of a token economy. The token economy should be simple and the "cost" of misbehavior should be posted as a visual reminder of the consequences of certain actions (e.g., hitting costs two tokens). Posting the consequences would also help the staff maintain consistency. At the end of the day children with tokens left could buy prizes (such as a Pokemon card). Each day children in the classroom would begin anew with consequences experienced the same day as the behavior (present oriented).

Items G and I of Making Choices and Item B of Roles helped identify the need for Step 2 of the plan. Having Michael participate in social skills groups in the context of the classroom helped address Michael's need for development of appropriate social skills, and encouraged the rest of the students not to provoke or encourage Michael's maladaptive behavior. The social skills group should be fun and may consist of activities such as team social skills trivia, or relay races that emphasize teamwork.

Part 3 of the plan is intended to help Michael expand his limited number of roles to include more functional roles and to help Michael practice transitioning from one role to another. Lunch and breakfast are served in the classroom in the Before and After School program and Michael regularly asked if he could help serve, but was not allowed to do so because it was more efficient for the staff to do it themselves. It was suggested that Michael be allowed to help serve one meal, either breakfast or lunch, on a regular basis. This would help him assume the functional role of classroom helper, and allow him to practice transitioning from a helper role when he is serving to a student/classmate role when he is eating with his peers.

The fourth step of the plan was proposed to help make transitions easier for Michael and the classroom staff. Items D and E of Making Choices and Item G of Habits and Routines helped to identify transitions as difficult for Michael. By preparing Michael in advance for coming transitions it will allow him to prepare himself and should lessen the number of cues that he currently requires during transitions.

The last step in Michael's plan to formally evaluate his fine and gross motor skills was included because, during the observations required for the scoring of the OT PAL, Michael exhibited difficulty in these areas. In games and craft activities that required more developed motor skills he often showed more frustration and quit sooner than expected with more claims that the activity was "stupid." The further development of Michael's fine and gross motor skills would allow Michael to more fully participate in activities with his peers and help to improve his self-concept.

Though it was clear that Michael needed some type of assistance to successfully function in the classroom, the OT PAL helped to identify the specific areas of concern in both the student and the environment. Michael's specific psychosocial and motor development needs, once met, may help reduce the barriers Michael faces in achieving success in the classroom and in life.

CONCLUSION

It is unfortunate that the topic of domestic violence ever has to be addressed. Life for children would be better if they never had to witness domestic violence and better still if the violence never occurred. The unfortunate reality is that it does occur and children who witness domestic violence, even if they are not abused themselves, are greatly affected by it. Occupational therapists can play a vital role in serving both the survivors and child witnesses of domestic violence. Occupational therapy with survivors and child witnesses of domestic violence may include developing skills needed for successful role performance, independent living skills, environmental adaptations, exploration of new roles, educational, prevocational, or vocational treatment (Helfrich, Lafata, LaEace-MacDonald, Aviles, & Collins, 2001). Additionally, as seen in this case study, occupational therapists have a role in assessing the classroom environment and how that environment meets the special needs of a child who has witnessed domestic violence.

This case study illustrates use of the OT PAL in a non-traditional classroom setting. In this case study, the OT PAL was valuable for identifying specific areas of concern within the environment and areas of psychosocial dysfunction in the child's school performance. The tool can be used with a variety of diagnoses and is designed for assessment of any child who is experiencing difficulty meeting the functional expectations of the classroom.

Areas for further research include determination of the long-term effects of witnessing domestic violence on children's volition and role functioning as they age. Longitudinal research is also needed to determine the long-term effects of occupational therapy intervention in working with child witnesses of domestic violence and the influence intervention has in ending the cycle of violence. Additionally, research to further explore gender differences in behavior patterns between witnesses of domestic violence would help those working in this field better serve these children.

REFERENCES

Fantuzzo, J., DePaola, L., Lambert, L., Martino, T., Anderson, G., & Sutton, S. (1991). Effects of interpersonal violence on the psychological adjustment and competencies of young children. *Journal of Consulting and Clinical Psychology*, 59(2), 258-265.

Helfrich, C. (2000). Domestic violence: Implications and guidelines for occupational therapy practitioners. In Cottrell, R.P. (Ed). *Proactive Approaches in Psychosocial Occupational Therapy*. Thorofare, NJ: Slack, 309-318.

Helfrich, C., Lafata, M., LaEace-MacDonald, S., Aviles, A., & Collins, L. (2001). Domestic abuse across the lifespan: Definitions, identification and risk factors for occupational therapists. *Occupational Therapy in Mental Health*, 16(3/4), 15-34.

Hughs, H. & Barad, S. (1983). Psychological functioning of children in a battered women's shelter: A preliminary investigation. *American Journal of Orthopsychiatry*, 53(3), 525-530.

Jaffe, P., Wolfe, D., & Wilson, S. (1990). *Children of Battered Women*. Newbury Park, CA: Sage.

Kielhofner, G. (1995). *A Model of Human Occupation: Theory and Practice.* (2nd ed.). Baltimore: Williams & Wilkins.

Kolbo, J., Blakley, E., & Engleman, D. (1996). Children who witness domestic violence: A review of empirical literature. *Journal of Interpersonal Violence,* 11(2), 281-293.

Nelms, B. (1994). Domestic violence: Children are victims too! *Journal of Pediatric Health Care,* 8, 201-202.

Thormaehlen, D. & Bass-Feld, E. (1994). Children: The secondary victims of domestic violence. *Maryland Medical Journal,* 43(4), 355-359.

Townsend, S., Carey, P., Hollins, N., Helfrich, C., Blondis, M., Hoffman, A., Collins, L., & Blackwell, A. (2000). *The Occupational Psychosocial Assessment of Learning.* Chicago, IL: Model of Human Occupation Clearinghouse, Department of Occupational Therapy, University of Illinois at Chicago.

APPENDIX

OCCUPATIONAL THERAPY PSYCHOSOCIAL ASSESSMENT OF LEARNING (O.T. PAL)

STUDENT _Michael_ DATE(S) _July 18, 2000 and July 26, 2000_
DATE OF BIRTH _02-27-82_ GRADE _2nd_ SCHOOL _Before and After_
TEACHER _Ms. Randolph_ OCCUPATIONAL THERAPIST _Jonathan Nave (OTS)_

The Occupational Therapy Psychosocial Assessment of Learning is a criterion-referenced rating scale and interview for use with children ages 6-12 years. It is designed for use within a school-based setting. Please refer to the manual for administration and scoring procedures. The rating scale is designed to be completed by an occupational therapist, with any behaviors not observed marked N/O. Teacher input via interview is expected to provide information on any areas not observed. Please refer to the specific rating scales located in the back of the manual for clarification of items.

Rating scale: N/O = not observed (activities observed did not require this), 1 = rarely or never observed (0-25 % of time required), 2 = occasionally (26-50% required), 3 = frequently (51-75% of time required), 4 = consistently (76-100% of time required)

I. Making Choices–Student chooses to:					
A. Begin an activity when given directions by an adult. Comments: *Requires several cues and often physical guidance*	N/O	1	②	3	4
B. Begin an activity in a self-directed manner when appropriate. Comments: *Consistently must be asked to clear table after lunch*	N/O	1	②	3	4
C. Stay engaged throughout an activity; continue to expend effort to complete it. Comments: *Usually will finish Uno game before beginning another play activity*	N/O	1	2	③	4
D. Continue with activity or transition to new activity when given directions by an adult. Comments:	N/O	1	②	3	4
E. Discontinue an activity when given directions by an adult. Comments: *Requires several verbal cues*	N/O	1	②	3	4
F. Discontinue an activity in a self-directed manner when appropriate. Comments: *Student rarely stops an activity unless he is asked to do so or he stops inappropriately*	N/O	①	2	3	4
G. Engage in activity/conversation within a peer group when given directions by an adult. Comments: *Must be cued as to appropriate conversation topic several times*	N/O	1	②	3	4
H. Engage in activity/conversation within a peer group in a self directed manner when appropriate. Comments: *Often enters conversations by yelling*	N/O	1	②	3	4
I. Follow social rules (e.g., sharing materials, taking turns). Comments: *Student has a hard time controlling himself, spends a significant amount of time being reprimanded*	N/O	①	2	3	4
J. Show preferences (likes/dislikes) for activities. Comments:	N/O	1	2	③	4

Section Total = 20/40

APPENDIX (continued)

II. Habits and Routines–The student:

A. Demonstrates school routines at a rate comparable to peers. Comments:	N/O	1	②	3	4
B. Adheres to routines within the school day. Comments: *Properly follows classroom routine of hanging up* *coat and backpack but must be reminded to sit down*	N/O	1	②	3	4
C. Completes activities within time guidelines (e.g., finishes assignments/tasks in a timely manner). Comments:	N/O	1	2	③	4
D. Maintains in a manner in keeping with classroom routines. Comments: *No personal desk in classroom*	Ⓝ/Ⓞ	1	2	3	4
E. Maintains personal belongings in keeping with classroom routines. Comments:	N/O	1	2	3	④
F. Organizes assignments and projects in keeping with classroom routines. Comments:	N/O	1	2	③	4
G. Completes smooth transitions between routine activities (i.e., efficiently ends and begins another). Comments: *90% of time the student had to be told repeatedly to* *stop an activity. Once stopped often began inappropriate activity*	N/O	①	2	3	4

Section Total =   15/24

III. Roles–The student:

A. Demonstrates a well-established student role (i.e., accepts teacher's authority, asks for help appropriately). Comments:	N/O	1	②	3	4
B. Demonstrates smooth transition between roles (i.e., switches smoothly from leader to follower). Comments: *When playing Uno often allowed peers to play for* *him (difficulty switching to self directed role)*	N/O	1	②	3	4
C. Responds acceptably to diverse roles adopted by others. Comments: *Much difficulty accepting teacher as* *playmate and authority*	N/O	①	2	3	4
D. Assumes roles consistent with classroom/school expectations. Comments: *Consistently falls into the same dysfunctional role* *(limited roles)*	N/O	①	2	3	4

Section Total =   6/16

APPENDIX (continued)

NARRATIVE REPORTS

Teacher Narrative:

a. Teacher's description of the classroom environment and his/her teaching style:
Teacher describes the classroom environment as relaxed with lots of free play activities into which she tries to incorporate communication and thinking skills as well as conflict resolution.
Teacher describes her teaching style as child directed. She is open to letting the children make some choices and decisions. And she states that she wants to make classroom activities fun.

b. Teacher's perspective of student's ability to meet classroom expectations:
Teacher states that Michael has a lot of potential, he just needs a lot of attention right now. Teacher believes that with time and a lot of work and attention Michael will be able to meet the classroom expectations. Currently the teacher believes that Michael knows the rules and classroom expectations but is unable to control his impulses and manage his anger enough to meet the expectations of the classroom.

c. Teacher's phrase to describe the student (i.e., "This child is . . ."):
Michael is a whiner, always negative, and never positive.

Student Narrative:

a. Student's description of the classroom (environment, routines, etc.):
Student was able to state several rules of the classroom, and stated that he had no special classroom jobs. Michael stated that he did not like the Before and After School Program because "there are too many rules and they never make pizza for lunch." Michael stated that he would rather work in groups, but was unable to identify anyone in the Before and After School Program that he liked being around except fictional (Pokemon) characters.

b. Student's narrative of him- or herself as a student and his/her ability to meet classroom expectations:
Student stated that he did not follow rules and when asked if he ever followed rules he said "no." He was not able to explain why. Michael also stated he did not have any friends in the class and he did not like the other kids (he specifically identified one child he did not like). He stated he was good at math and writing. Michael explained that when he grows up he would like to be a policeman because, "they have handcuffs and guns and got to shoot gang bangers and other people."

Parent's Narrative:

Mother reported that Michael did not talk about the Before and After School Program much at home, but believed that he did not like the program because he has trouble following the rules and was often in trouble. The mother reported that her son had a very positive attitude and named 2 other children in the classroom that Michael really liked (one of the children was the child Michael specifically identified as not liking). The mother stated she believed that Michael knows what the classroom rules are and how to follow them, but that he has always had a hard time in academic settings. She stated that she believed that Michael liked the Before and After School Program.

APPENDIX (continued)

SUMMARY/ASSESSMENT

Scores (average of items observed):

Making Choices	<u>20/40</u>
Habits & Routines	<u>15/24</u>
Roles	<u>6/16</u>
Total Score	<u>41/80</u>

Student/Environment Fit:

The environment meets Michael's needs by providing clearly defined rules and expectations. The staff attempts to meet Michael's need for one-on-one assistance, although that need is not always met. The classroom provides many opportunities for Michael to develop appropriate social skills and assume functional roles. Additionally, the classroom staff provides activities that are both challenging and fun.

The environment does not meet Michael's need for structure and is often too disordered for Michael to attend to tasks and activities. Other students in the classroom also interfere with Michael's ability to function by sometimes provoking and encouraging his maladaptive behavior. The consequences for Michael's behavior are not always consistent, and often involve taking away privileges too far in the future for Michael's present-oriented thinking.

Summary of Strengths and Needs:

Strengths	Needs
Michael's strengths: Desire to participate in most classroom activities, inquisitive, likes to laugh and have a good time. *Classroom strengths:* Teacher is open to new ideas, many opportunities for students to participate in class activities, environment allows for choice and self-direction by the students.	Michael needs clear rules and structure to function at his best. Limited roles, needs to have structured opportunity to acquire new role to build self-esteem and increase functional roles. Michael's social competence is poor and he would benefit from social skills education to help him learn how to respond and act appropriately with peers and adults. During therapist's observation of Michael fine and gross motor activities seemed to be problematic for Michael. NEED: Formal evaluation of motor skills and determination of eligibility for school system services in occupational and physical therapy.

APPENDIX (continued)

Intervention Plan:

Recommendations to be implemented by classroom staff:
1. *Develop a behavioral control plan that is consistent and present oriented.*
2. *Encourage Michael to participate in group activities that emphasize social skills education.*
3. *Help Michael develop functional roles by including him in activities such as serving lunch, or passing out supplies.*
4. *Begin giving Michael time warnings that an activity will be ending soon (e.g., "Michael in ten minutes you will need to put up the paints you are using." Five minutes later, "Michael you have five more minutes to finish up.").*

Further need for clinical intervention:
5. *Formally evaluate Michael's fine and gross motor skills.*

The Occupational Therapy Elder Abuse Checklist

Mary Jean Lafata, MS, OTR/L
Christine A. Helfrich, PhD, OTR/L

SUMMARY. Occupational therapists encounter elder abuse in society and in clinical practice; however, the occupational therapy literature is void of information and tools for assessing and treating individuals at risk. Occupational therapists are in a unique position to identify elder abuse. Definitions of elder abuse, signs and symptoms of elder abuse, and reporting practices required of professionals coming in contact with individuals who may have been abused are presented. The Occupational Therapy Elder Abuse Checklist was developed to assist the occupational therapist as well as other health care professionals in uncovering abusive situations of elders who are either living alone or living with others. Guidelines are provided for use with the tool. A case study illustrates use of the tool for reporting suspected abuse, and the assessment and treatment of an individual who is a victim of elder abuse. *[Article copies available for a fee from The Haworth Document Delivery Service: 1-800-342-9678. E-mail address: <getinfo@haworthpressinc.com> Website: <http://www.HaworthPress.com> © 2001 by The Haworth Press, Inc. All rights reserved.]*

KEYWORDS. Elder abuse, neglect, occupational therapy assessment

Mary Jean Lafata is an Occupational Therapy Manager (E-mail: *mlafatal@aol.com*).

Christine A. Helfrich is Assistant Professor, Department of Occupational Therapy, University of Illinois at Chicago, 1919 W. Taylor Street (M/C 811), Chicago, IL 60612 (E-mail: *Helfrich@uic.edu*).

For questions pertaining to this article, please direct all correspondence to Dr. Christine Helfrich.

[Haworth co-indexing entry note]: "The Occupational Therapy Elder Abuse Checklist." Lafata, Mary Jean, and Christine A. Helfrich. Co-published simultaneously in *Occupational Therapy in Mental Health* (The Haworth Press, Inc.) Vol. 16, No. 3/4, 2001, pp. 141-161; and: *Domestic Abuse Across the Lifespan: The Role of Occupational Therapy* (ed: Christine A. Helfrich) The Haworth Press, Inc., 2001, pp. 141-161. Single or multiple copies of this article are available for a fee from The Haworth Document Delivery Service [1-800-342-9678, 9:00 a.m. - 5:00 p.m. (EST). E-mail address: getinfo@haworthpressinc.com].

INTRODUCTION

Every occupational therapy evaluation of the elderly client in any setting should include an assessment of the possibility of abuse occurring to that client. It has been estimated that 5% of the elderly population, or more than 1 million elders, are abused annually (U.S. Congress, 1990). The oldest elders in our population (age 80 and over) are abused and neglected at two to three times their proportion of the elderly population (National Center on Elder Abuse, 1998). Elder abuse often goes unreported, with estimates that only one in eight cases is reported to authorities (Larue, 1992; U.S. Congress, 1990). Estimates of the incidence and prevalence of abuse and neglect vary considerably. It is difficult to compare results across various studies directly because of significant differences in research definitions, objectives, and methodologies.

A random sample community based epidemiological study of abuse investigating 2020 Boston area adults 65 years or older was conducted (Pillemer, K. & Finkelhor, D., 1988). The elders were asked about three forms of maltreatment: physical violence, psychological abuse, and neglect. Of the sample surveyed, 3.2% reported having experienced some form of maltreatment since they turned 65 years old. In the study, physical abuse emerged as the predominant type of abuse suffered (2.2%) followed by habitual verbal aggression (1.1%) and neglect (0.4%) (Pillemer & Finkelhor, 1988). The low rate of neglect most likely reflects the narrow definitions of abuse used by the researchers. Another study indicated that women are victims of 75% of the incidents of psychological abuse and 92% of financial abuse/exploitation cases (Butler, 1999).

DEFINITIONS OF ELDER ABUSE

Physical Abuse

Physical abuse is violence that results in bodily harm, or a means of inflicting physical pain or injury upon the elder. Physical abuse may include but is not limited to acts of violence such as: striking with or without an object, hitting, beating, pushing, shoving, shaking, slapping, kicking, pinching, and burning. The unwarranted administration of drugs and physical restraints, force feeding, and physical punishment of any kind are also examples of physical abuse.

Financial Abuse/Exploitation

Financial abuse/exploitation is the misuse or misappropriation of the elder's money or assets that results in a disadvantage to the elder and/or the profit of someone else. Examples include: being forced to turn over money or property, forging an elder's signature, misusing or stealing an elder's money or possessions, coercing or deceiving an elder into signing a document, and the improper use of guardianship, conservatorship, or power of attorney.

Emotional/Psychological Abuse

Emotional/psychological abuse is an act carried out with the intention of causing emotional pain or injury. Emotional or psychological abuse includes but is not limited to verbal assaults, insults, threats, intimidation, humiliation, and embarrassment. In addition, treating an elder like an infant; isolating an elder from family, friends or regular activities; giving an elder the "silent treatment"; and enforced social isolation are examples of emotional and/or psychological abuse.

Sexual Abuse

Sexual abuse is an act of forced sexual intimacy or any nonconsensual sexual contact of any kind with an elder. Sexual contact with any person who is unable to consent is also considered sexual abuse and touching, fondling or any other sexual activity with an elder, when the person is unable to understand, unwilling to consent, threatened, or physically forced. Examples include but are not limited to: unwanted touching, all types of sexual assault or battery such as rape, sodomy, coerced nudity, and sexually explicit photographing.

Neglect

Neglect is the caregiver's failure to provide the elder with life's necessities. The neglect may be intentional, when a caregiver deliberately fails his/her responsibilities in order to punish the elder. Examples include willfully withholding medicine, food, or water. The neglect may also be unintentional, resulting from ignorance or a genuine inability to complete the task. Examples include: not changing an elder's diaper frequently enough resulting in decubitus ulcers or being forcibly confined or restrained. Self-neglect is defined as an elder withholding food, medicine, medical treatment or personal care necessary for his or her well-being. Examples include not taking prescribed medications or refusing medical treatment.

Abandonment

Abandonment is the desertion of an elderly person by an individual who has assumed responsibility for providing care or by a person with physical custody of an elder.

Violation of Rights

All Americans are gifted with certain inalienable rights by the U.S. Constitution and federal and state laws. Examples of violation of rights include: being forced out of one's home or being forced into another setting without due process, being deprived of the right to move freely without physical restraints, being deprived of adequate and appropriate medical treatment, having one's property taken without due process of law, being deprived of a clean and safe environment, having the right to privacy denied, or being deprived of freedom from verbal abuse. The right to complain or have grievances addressed is also an inalienable right (U.S. Congress, 1990). In addition to these rights, according to Quinn and Tomita (1986), violation of rights includes being denied the right or opportunity to vote, attend church, or open one's own personal mail. Denial or violation of these rights is a form of abuse, which is reportable. Many of these rights are also included in other definitions of abuse mentioned above.

Problems with Defining Abuse

Many of the problems with defining abuse focus on the issue of neglect. Neglect of the elderly raises difficult questions such as: Who is the responsible party or caretaker? What are their responsibilities? Was the neglect intentional or unintentional? The final result of neglect is the breakdown of the elder's ability to survive in the community. The first intervention should be directed at improving function and quality of life and allowing the elder to live in the community with minimal assistance, instead of looking to assign blame for the situation. To avoid assigning blame for the situation many authorities prefer to avoid the terms "abuse" or "neglect" and use phrases such as "inadequate care of the elderly" or "mistreatment of the elderly," which includes acts of both omission and commission (Fulmer & O'Malley, 1987; Johnson, 1991). However, the lack of forthright definitions works to minimize the problem of elder abuse. (See Table 1.)

ELDER ABUSE SCREENING TOOLS

The Elder Abuse Checklist was developed to assist health care professionals in uncovering abuse in the elderly population. There is

TABLE 1. Signs and Symptoms of Abuse and Neglect

Type of Abuse	Indicator of Abuse
Physical Abuse (King & Ryan, 1989; Moss & Taylor, 1991; National Center on Elder Abuse, 1998)	■ Bruises in unusual places (back of arm, breast or genitals), bruises at various stages of healing (indicating repetitive pattern of injury), welts, black eyes, untreated injuries, open wounds, punctures. ■ Burns caused by cigarettes, ropes, "dry burns" caused by irons or stoves, particularly in unusual places (the back) or of prolonged severity. ■ Lacerations to the facial area (lips, eyes) or genitals. ■ Orthopedic Injuries that do not fit the individual's developmental level or explanation (spiral fracture to the arm explained by falling down stairs), strains and/or dislocations. ■ Head & facial injuries such as subdural hematomas (caused by shaking or hitting), absence of hair, retinal and jaw injuries, skull fractures. ■ Internal injuries including injury to an unborn fetus caused by external trauma to the stomach area. ■ Broken eyeglasses/frames, physical signs of being subjected to punishment or signs of being restrained. ■ Laboratory findings of medical overdose or underutilization of prescribed medications. ■ Reports of being slapped or mistreated. ■ Sudden change of behavior. ■ Refusal of the caregiver to allow visitors to see the dependent alone.

TABLE 1 (continued)

Type of Abuse	Indicator of Abuse
Sexual Abuse (National Center on Elder Abuse, 1998)	▪ Bruises around the breast or genital area. ▪ Unexplained venereal disease or genital infections. ▪ Unexplained vaginal or anal bleeding. ▪ Torn, stained or bloody underclothing. ▪ Being sexually assaulted or raped.
Emotional/Psychological Abuse (National Center on Elder Abuse, 1998)	▪ Emotional upset or agitation. ▪ Extreme withdrawal and non-communicative or non-responsiveness. ▪ Being verbally or emotionally mistreated.
Neglect (National Center on Elder Abuse, 1998)	▪ Dehydration, malnutrition, untreated bedsores and/or poor personal hygiene. ▪ Unattended or untreated health problems. ▪ Hazardous or unsafe living conditions. ▪ Unsanitary or unclean living conditions. ▪ A dependent's report of being neglected.
Self-neglect (National Center on Elder Abuse, 1998)	▪ Dehydration, malnutrition, untreated or improperly attended medical conditions, and poor personal hygiene. ▪ Hazardous or unsafe living conditions. ▪ Unsanitary or unclean living conditions. ▪ Inappropriate and/or inadequate clothing, lack of necessary medical aids. ▪ Grossly inadequate housing or homelessness.
Abandonment (National Center on Elder Abuse, 1998)	▪ The desertion of a dependent at a hospital, nursing facility or other similar institution. ▪ The desertion of a dependent at a shopping mall or other public location. ▪ A dependent's own report of being abandoned.
Financial or Material Exploitation (National Center on Elder Abuse, 1998)	▪ Sudden changes in a bank account or banking practice, including an unexplained withdrawal of large sums of money by a person accompanying the elder. ▪ The inclusion of additional names on an elder's bank signature card. ▪ Unauthorized withdrawal of funds using an elder's ATM card. ▪ Abrupt changes in a will or other financial documents. ▪ Unexplained disappearance of funds or valuable possessions. ▪ Provisions of substandard care or bills unpaid despite the availability of adequate funds. ▪ The provision of services that are not necessary. ▪ Discovery of an elder's signature forged for financial transactions or for the titles of the elder's possessions. ▪ Sudden appearance of previously uninvolved relatives claiming rights to an elder's affairs and possessions. ▪ Unexplained sudden transfer of assets to a family member or someone outside of the family. ▪ An elder's report of financial exploitation.

currently little occupational therapy literature on the subject of elder abuse. In a review of occupational therapy literature under the description of elder abuse, one article was uncovered. This article, entitled *Ethical Dilemmas in Family Caregiving for the Elderly: Implications for Occupational Therapy*, did not deal directly with abuse of the elderly; instead ethical dilemmas in care for the elderly were discussed (Hasselkus, 1991). A careful review of health care literature revealed that several instruments have been developed to assess elder abuse in the medical and nursing fields. More research needs to be completed to determine their usefulness in assisting nurses and other professionals involved with elders in uncovering elder abuse. The following assessment tools are noted because they represent those most frequently cited in the review of literature for elder abuse.

The High-Risk Placement Worksheet (HRPW)

The High-Risk Placement Worksheet (HRPW) was designed to assess the quantitative and qualitative characteristics of the elder, major caregiver, and family system. This assessment was designed to signal potential abuse related to the characteristics of the elder and caregiver. In this assessment, which is used like a checklist, the examiner evaluates whether or not there is an existence of risk for the characteristics of the elder, the caregiver or the family system. The congruity of perceptions from the elder and caregiver are compared to assess if there is a difference present. If there is incongruity, the evaluation determines if this difference constitutes a risk for the elder.

The Health Status, Attitudes Toward Aging, Living Arrangements, and Finances

The Health Status, Attitudes Toward Aging, Living Arrangements and Finances (HALF) assesses four factors contributing to elder abuse to determine risk and the appropriate interventions. In each area described above, the HALF uses a checklist format. Almost always, some of the time, and never are the responses, and risk is determined according to the views the examiner has of the client and caregiver. It is important to state that the presence of some or all of the characteristics or factors in these checklists is not necessarily indicative of an abusive situation and should not automatically be construed as such.

Additional instruments have been designed to discover elder abuse within the home. Those instruments cited most frequently in the literature on elder abuse include The Elderly Assessment Protocol (TEAP) (Haviland, 1989; Hamilton, 1989), Vulnerability Assessment Score of Aged Persons (VASAP) (Haviland, 1989; Hamilton, 1989), Stress Assessment Score of the Caregiver (SASC) (Haviland, 1989; Hamilton, 1989), and the Risk of Elder Abuse in the Home (REAH) (Haviland, 1989; Hamilton, 1989). Further information on the validity and reliability of all these assessments is needed (Hamilton, 1989).

Many professionals also rely on their own interview techniques rather than use of a tool; however, the use of an assessment instrument or tool aids the health care provider by providing a systematic assessment, as well as data for use in documentation.

Occupational Therapy Elder Abuse Checklist

In response to this lack of available occupational therapy tools to assess elder abuse, the Occupational Therapy Elder Abuse Checklist was developed in two versions: (1) Elders who live alone, and (2) Elders who live with others. Guidelines (Table 2) were developed to assist the professional in completing a thorough evaluation using the checklists to aid in uncovering possible abuse or neglect to a client. An example of a completed checklist is provided in Figure 1: Mrs. A, Occupational Therapy Elder Abuse Checklist.

The checklists are designed to assist the professional in completing a thorough evaluation and in uncovering possible abuse or neglect to a client. Checklist items allow the professional to understand certain aspects of the elder's care (i.e., who is responsible for medications, medical appointments, and the elder's basic needs). Suggested questions in the guidelines provide a basis for exploring exactly whom the elder comes into contact with daily and the attitudes of those individuals toward the elder. Both the elder and the caregiver answer the same questions. This provides the therapist with a mechanism to compare the elder and the caregiver's perceptions of the home environment.

CASE STUDY

The following is a case study of a client seen by the author in a home setting.

TABLE 2. Guide for Completing the Elder Abuse Checklist

Issue	Sample Questions (to be tailored to elder's environment)
Health Issues	1. Do you understand why your mother is taking the following medications? List the medications. 2. Your mother has just had hip replacement surgery; are you aware of the precautions of movement after this surgery? 3. Your father has a sore on his back; do you understand the importance of keeping him from lying prolonged on his back? 4. Who makes the doctor appointments? 5. How did you break your arm? This question should be asked in private. 6. How did your mother break her arm? This question should be asked in private. 7. How is your vision, hearing, or memory? Do you forget medications or doctor appointments? Same questions to the caregiver.
Caregiver Attitudes	1. Do you feel comfortable with all the aspects of your father's care? 2. What are you having difficulty with? 3. It can be very difficult dealing with an older person. Do you have help to relieve you? 4. How are you feeling? Do you feel sad or blue a lot? If so, have you ever been hospitalized for this? 5. Do you and your husband see eye to eye on most issues that affect his care? 6. How do you get along with your mother? 7. Caregiving can be a difficult task. How do you feel about being the primary caregiver? Do you ever feel trapped? 8. Caregiving can be a difficult task. How do you unwind? Do you drink alcohol or smoke cigarettes? How often do you do this?
Financial Issues	1. Does your mother have adequate resources to provide for her needs? 2. Do you (the caregiver) have an income aside from your father's income? 3. Ask the client. Do you feel your caregiver adequately uses your resources? 4. Who writes your checks and pays your bills? 5. Are you comfortable with this financial situation? 6. Do you know how, where, and when your money is spent?
Support Systems for Caregiver and/or Client	1. Do you see your family and friends often? 2. Is help close by when you need it? 3. Who do you call for help? 4. Would you have to wait a long time for assistance? 5. Would you like to have a *Lifeline* installed in your home to assist with calling for help if you were unable to reach the phone? (Lifeline is a commercial product that contacts a series of people (family, neighbors, 911) designated by the elder, in case of emergency.) 6. Who do you talk to when you are upset? (Question for either client or caregiver)

TABLE 2 (continued)

Issue	Sample Questions (to be tailored to elder's environment)
	7. Is Mrs. L. fair in her treatment of you? (Ask privately to both client and caregiver.) 8. Are you happy with your current living situation? (Ask the client) 9. Are you ever afraid of your caregiver? 10. Does your caregiver yell at you? 11. Have you ever been hit or slapped? 12. Would you like a Senior Citizens Resource Guide that points out all the services available to the elderly and disabled in this area?
Safety Issues	1. Show me how you get into the tub? On the toilet? 2. Do you have difficulty getting dressed? Has anyone ever suggested a reacher, sock donner, etc.? 3. Who takes you shopping? 4. Do you pay them to take you shopping? How much? Do you feel this is reasonable? 5. Have you ever been physically hurt by anyone? 6. Have you ever been threatened by anyone? 7. Do you feel safe at home? 8. Do you feel you could use some help keeping your home clean? 9. Do you have trouble negotiating around the rooms in your home? Does your walker fit through the doors? Are there things that could be moved to make it safer for you to move around your home?

Background Information

Mrs. A (all names have been changed for anonymity) was a 76-year-old female with a diagnosis of osteoarthritis and coronary artery disease (CAD). Mrs. A lived with two of her daughters; one of her daughters owned the home in which she lived. Mrs. A came to live with her daughter 2 years ago as a result of her inability to live alone due to fear of falling. The daughter's home was a 3-bedroom split level ranch with 9 stairs up to the bedrooms from the living room, the kitchen and eating area on the main level, and 6 stairs down to the family room and a half bath. There were no bathroom facilities on the main level where Mrs. A spent the majority of her day. This required her to go up and down at least 6 stairs to go to the bathroom. Mrs. A was taking diuretics prescribed by her physician and needed to use the bathroom 5-7 times a day.

Referral

Mrs. A was referred for home health occupational therapy services from her family physician as a result of a recent hospitalization for

CAD. Her family was complaining that she was unable to take care of her basic needs for 3-4 months prior to her hospitalization.

Evaluation

During the initial evaluation, Mrs. A stated that she would like to be able to complete her activities of daily living skills independently as she had 4 months prior. Mrs. A also wished to be able to make a light meal using the microwave, if necessary. Mrs. A was motivated to work and had a positive outlook on her prognosis. She requested a home exercise program almost immediately upon completion of the evaluation. Mrs. A enjoyed the company of others and belonged to several senior groups in her area.

Mrs. A described a gradual loss of independence over a 4-5 month period of time. She stated that she began to notice weaknesses 4-5 months prior to hospitalization; however, her physician dismissed it as "the normal aging process." Mrs. A stated that her daughter resented having to help her from the beginning; when she felt too weak to get into the shower, her daughter would call her "lazy." As the weeks went on she was unable to dress herself independently and finally she needed assistance with getting onto the toilet. At this point her daughter took her to the doctor and insisted that the physician "find out what was wrong with her." Mrs. A was hospitalized for 3 days and released to her home with home health care services to provide the nursing and rehabilitation that she had previously received as an inpatient at a rehabilitation center during one of her previous hospitalizations.

Mrs. A presented with moderate deficits in activities of daily living. Oral/facial hygiene was completed independently by Mrs. A following set up of a basin with water and all needed equipment such as toothbrush, toothpaste and washcloth. She was unable to transfer into the shower or onto the toilet independently. Bathing was completed with the assistance of 1 person at the bedside, as Mrs. A was unable to stand in the shower independently. She required the assistance of 1 person for transfer due to balance and lower extremity weakness problems. Mrs. A was able to complete all hygiene tasks associated with toileting independently. Moving from sitting to standing required the assistance of 1 person. Mrs. A was unable to dress herself independently. She was able to put on her brassiere and shirt independently, but was unable to get her pants or socks over her feet or pull them up to her waist due to balance and lower extremity strength problems. In addition, Mrs. A required assistance for meal preparation. Some areas of her kitchen were inaccessible in her wheelchair, including some cabinets where the food was located. The only cleaning tasks Mrs. A was able to complete from her wheelchair were making her bed, loading the dishwasher, and dusting her bedroom.

Mrs. A stated that she was frustrated and felt like a burden to her daughter, with whom she was living. She felt the need to increase her independence as soon as possible. There was an urgency to her tone that cued the therapist to further explore her difficulties. When asked about her finances and the possibility of obtaining household help, she stated that it would be necessary to talk with her daughter concerning monetary issues.

After completing the evaluation (and obtaining Mrs. A's permission) the therapist spoke with her daughter to ascertain her opinion of her mother's functioning, to gain more insight into the financial aspects of acquiring help in the home, and to evaluate the daughter's (caregiver's) response to the difficulties Mrs. A was experiencing. Upon interviewing Mrs. A's daughter (Marge), the therapist found her to be quite angry with her mother. She blamed her mother for her recent loss of function and insinuated that she was purposefully not completing her ADL independently because she liked the attention and it was easier to let others do things for her. She stated that she felt both overwhelmed and depressed in caring for her mother. Marge stated that she felt "no joy" in being with her mother anymore and needed help as soon as possible. Marge stated that Mrs. A had adequate monetary resources to pay for help, but she was reluctant to hire someone to care for her mother as she feared that she would become more dependent and she did not like the idea of "another person" being in her home.

With the initial evaluation completed, the therapist decided it was necessary to complete the Occupational Therapy Elder Abuse Checklist: Lives with Others, and further explore the possibility of whether elder abuse might be occurring in the family (please refer to Figure 1). Occupational therapy lends itself well to identifying elder abuse. In evaluating activities of daily living there are ample opportunities to discover elder abuse that may be occurring. Bruises may be discovered, lack of adequate nutrition or medications may be evident, neglect may be apparent, or verbal abuse may be detected. It may be necessary to contact other team members to ascertain their thoughts and impres-

FIGURE 1. Mrs. A: Occupational Therapy Elder Abuse Checklist

O.T. Elder Abuse Checklist Elder Lives with Others			
Client Name: Mrs. A **Primary Caregiver:** Daughter **Age:** 76 **Description of Living Situation:** 3 bedroom ranch with stairs			
	Yes	**No**	**Unsure**
Health Issues			
Is family/caregiver aware of medical needs?	√		
Is family/caregiver aware of needed medications?	√		
Is family/caregiver aware of the elder's limitations?		√	
Does family/caregiver believe limitations are legitimate?		√	
Are injuries common with this client?		√	
Does the client present with unexplained injuries?		√	
Are accounts of injuries different from client and family/caregiver?		√	
Does family/caregiver assist client to keep/make Dr. appointments?	√		
Caregiver Attitudes/Problems			
Is there marital conflict between the client and spouse?			√
Does family/caregiver act appropriately with serious medical condition (Does not over/under react)?	√		
Does family/caregiver have problems with drugs/alcohol?		√	
Does family/caregiver have history of mental illness?		√	
Does family/caregiver appear depressed?	√		
Does family/caregiver feel "trapped" or burdened by client?	√		
Is family/caregiver openly hostile toward client?	√		
Is family/caregiver negative about the aging process?	√		
Is family/caregiver pleasant with client?		√	
Is family/caregiver unable (mentally/physically) or unwilling to meet client's needs?	√		
Is client pleasant with family/caregiver?	√		
Does client appear frightened or unusually quiet in the presence of family/caregiver?	√		
Finances			
Is family/caregiver reliant on client for income/housing/food?		√	
Does family/caregiver have financial difficulties?		√	
Is the client further burdening the family/caregiver with finances?		√	
Support Systems for Caregiver and/or Client			
Does family/caregiver have an adequate support system for their needs?		√	
Is the client burdening the family with overcrowding in the home?		√	
Does family/caregiver have adequate respite care from client?	√		
Does family/caregiver feel this is an adequate amount of time?		√	
Does client appear happy with current living situation?		√	
Is there a need for ADL equipment or resources?	√		
Observations/Perception			
1. What is the client's perception of the ideal living environment? **Somewhere I can be happy.**			
2. What is the family/caregiver response to ideal living environment? **Right here at home.**			
3. Is the therapist uncomfortable in any way with the current living situation for this client? **Yes.** If so, why? **Living situation stressful for all.**			
Number of visits used to complete this checklist: 1			

© Lafata, 2000

sions regarding the possibility of elder abuse. Team members include the nurse, home health aide, physical therapist, and the occupational therapist. In this case, the occupational therapist recommended a social work consultation since she found there was the possibility of elder abuse occurring with Mrs. A.

Occupational Therapy Elder Abuse Checklist Results

Health Issues

Mrs. A's daughter was aware of her medical and medication needs; however, she was unaware of her mother's limitations and was reluctant to believe the therapist's recommendations, as she felt the therapists were being misled by her mother. There was no evidence of physical abuse, and injuries were not common with this client. Marge made and kept all doctor appointments for her mother.

Caregiver Attitudes/Problems

There was no evidence of an over or under reaction to Mrs. A's medical conditions by her caregiver. There was no apparent history of mental illness or drug/alcohol abuse by Marge, although such information was not available to the team. Marge appeared depressed and overwhelmed at times. She was overtly hostile to her mother and stated that she felt burdened by her mother. Marge viewed aging from a negative perspective and required reminders of the positive aspects to aging, such as wisdom and patience. Marge was rarely pleasant with her mother when staff was present and when Mrs. A was asked if there were times that she and Marge got along she said, "no." The therapist felt as though Mrs. A did what she could to be pleasant with her daughter; however, this seemed to go unnoticed by Marge, who felt her mother did not like her. When asked to further explain, Marge stated that they never talk anymore. Mrs. A did appear very quiet in Marge's presence and allowed her to do most of the talking. Mrs. A told the therapist that she stayed quiet to avoid further disagreements with her daughter. When the therapist suggested to Marge that Mrs. A might be trying to avoid further possible disagreements with her, Marge became tearful. Mrs. A was asked if she felt afraid or frightened of her daughter at any time and she stated that she never felt her daughter would physically harm her, but she hurt her feelings many times a day.

Financial Issues

Marge was not reliant upon Mrs. A for support at any time. There were no apparent financial difficulties or trouble with finances in the home.

Support Systems for Caregiver and/or Client

There was no evidence of overcrowding in the home. There was not an adequate caregiver support system to meet Mrs. A's or Marge's needs. Mrs. A had another daughter who also lived in the home; however, that daughter was reluctant to offer any suggestions for the current situation because of her own reliance on her sister, Marge, for housing. There was no respite available to Marge, except for her sister who did not have a role in her mother's care except for occasionally "mother sitting" when Marge went out shopping. Neither Marge nor her mother was happy with their current living situation as both women became tearful when asked. Each woman was interviewed separately which allowed for freedom of true expression.

Observations/Perception

When Mrs. A was asked what her ideal living situation would be she stated, "Somewhere I can be happy." Marge's response to her mother's ideal living situation was "Right here at home." This living situation is stressful for all involved. There were obvious negative feelings between mother and daughter and between both sisters. Marge appears to be the dominant woman in the home and appears to control all events that happen in the home. For the reasons outlined above the therapist believed that Mrs. A was suffering from psychological and verbal abuse in her current living situation. It was not felt that Mrs. A was in imminent danger; therefore, all team members were consulted prior to confronting the family or reporting the abuse to the elder abuse hotline.

Team Involvement

All *team members* were contacted by voice mail and responded within 24 hours. Team members included the nurse, home health aide, occupational therapist, and physical therapist. The *nurse*, whose role was to monitor Mrs. A's vital signs, medications and provide instruction regarding the medications that were being used, noted a negative attitude toward the aging process by both Mrs. A and her daughter. She stated she felt that Marge was negative toward her mother, but was not sure if it was a daily problem or if she was just having a bad day. She stated she saw no signs of physical abuse, but agreed that there was a possibility of verbal and/or emotional abuse and agreed to further explore the issue on her next visit. Mrs. A's physician authorized the nurse to visit twice each week for 2 weeks.

The *home health aide*, whose role was to bathe the client, felt that there was inadequate respite for family members for daily care. She stated that Marge called her a "Godsend" and asked her how she could stand taking care of older people all day long. She stated that she felt that Mrs. A was being verbally abused. The home health aide was a valuable person to contact for corroboration of the team's findings because she also had intimate contact with the client and the ability to observe bruises or other skin problems that may occur as a result of abuse. The physician gave orders for the home health aide to visit Mrs. A 3 times per week for 6 weeks.

The *physical therapist's* goals were to assist Mrs. A with exercises to improve her strength and endurance, improve her balance in standing, and improve ambulation on stairs and flat surfaces. The physical therapist noted that Mrs. A's daughter was insisting that her mother be able to walk down 9 stairs to the kitchen area to complete her lunch time meal preparation independently and walk down 6 stairs to the bathroom to complete her toileting. Marge also commented that if her mother could not perform those tasks, she would put her in a nursing home. The physical therapist felt this was an unreasonable expectation at the time and informed Marge that it would be several weeks before this would happen if it were possible at all. The physical therapist also noted some "tension" between mother and daughter; Marge yelled at her mother to pay attention to the therapist and threatened to put her in a nursing home if she did not "do well" in therapy.

The *social worker's* role was to assist Mrs. A and her family in obtaining all needed social services. The social worker was able to ascertain that Mrs. A had adequate funds to afford further assistance in the home, but that her daughter was reluctant to have any more people assisting her mother, fearing that she would become completely dependent upon them. The social worker felt that anger management was a problem for Marge. Recommendations for agencies that provide daily care to the elderly were made. Recommendations were also made for Marge to attend a support group for caregivers and an anger management seminar.

All *team members* were asked in the telephone contacts if they felt Mrs. A was in an abusive situation and all agreed that she was. The team decided that the occupational therapist, who was the person with whom the abuse allegation originated, and the nurse, who was the case manager, would meet with the family to discuss the concerns. The team felt that there was no immediate danger for Mrs. A and that the situation could possibly be remedied with education, equipment, therapy services (continued occupational therapy and physical therapy services), respite care from friends in the community, and a daily part-time home health aide several hours a day. Therefore, the team decided to meet with the family before reporting the case to the Elder Abuse Hotline.

Elder Abuse Intervention

A meeting was scheduled to discuss the elder abuse allegations, the report to the elder abuse hotline, and the recommendations made by the team. Mrs. A, Marge, Mrs. A's other daughter, the nurse and the occupational therapist all met in Mrs. A's home. Marge was angered and embarrassed by the elder abuse allegation and proposed report, but eventually was able to understand the team's responsibility to Mrs. A's well being. The team informed the family that their assistance to Mrs. A included assistance and education to them as well and that the team's intention was not to destroy the family unit, but to provide some needed assistance to Mrs. A and her family. The goals of the meeting were to educate the family concerning elder abuse, provide Mrs. A's family with information concerning her current level of functioning, provide equipment and aide recommendations, and provide referrals for respite care. The team's agenda included education concerning Mrs. A's osteoarthritis, CAD, the aging process, and managing a disabled elder at home. The team recommended a part-time aide 4 hours a day to assist Mrs. A with her activities of daily living (ADL), and provide respite for her family. ADL equipment was also recommended to assist Mrs. A with completion of her ADL. A transfer tub bench for the bathtub, long-handled sponge, raised toilet seat with safety frames, a reacher, and elastic shoelaces were issued to assist with independent completion of ADL. The team suggested inviting some of Mrs. A's friends from the community as respite care. Mrs. A was very happy with all recommendations and appeared relieved that someone noticed and cared enough to address the issue. She stated that she felt as though she could confide in her health care providers and experienced an empowering situation in which she could take a more active role in her care. Mrs. A wanted to do more to relieve stress in the family.

Marge was hostile, angry, and in disagreement with the allegations and report to the hotline. She disagreed with the need for a part-time home health aide 4 hours per day, but was willing to try it out to see if it would work. Within days of receiving the equipment and training, having the home health aide 4 hours a day, and receiving occupational therapy and physical therapy 2-3 times a week, Mrs. A was functioning at minimal assistance for dressing and hygiene and was able to ascend 6 stairs with minimal to moderate assistance of 1 person. Mrs. A was happy with her therapy progress. Marge was also pleased with her progress, although she was anxious to decrease the time that the home health aide spent with her mother in her home.

After 6 weeks of therapy, Mrs. A was able to walk up 6 stairs with stand-by assistance for safety, shower with stand-by assistance for safety, and dress herself independently with the use of a reacher, long shoe horn and elastic shoelaces. She needed stand-by assistance to complete light cooking using the microwave and began to assist with light cleaning from the sitting position of her wheelchair.

CONCLUSIONS AND DISCUSSION

When an occupational therapist evaluates an individual, rapport is usually quickly established as a result of the personal questions asked and the nature of activities that must be observed. The therapist's tone of voice, mannerisms, and length of time spent with the client also assist in the establishment of rapport. Therefore, it is essential that occupational therapists represent themselves and the profession in a caring and thoughtful manner. There are times when home health care personnel are the only contacts with the outside world that an individual may have. It is imperative that occupational therapists are thorough, kind, and honest in their evaluations and recommendations for individuals.

It can be difficult to make judgments concerning elder abuse in a client's home. As mandated reporters for elders who are unable to report for themselves, the answer is simple. A mandated reporter must report any form of abuse to the elder abuse hotline. When an elder is able to report for him or herself the line becomes fuzzy. There is no legal act requiring a professional to report; however, voluntary reporting is very much encouraged. In physical abuse cases it is much easier to make a decision to call the elder abuse hotline; however, when emotional or psychological abuse is suspected there may be reluctance to involve the authorities. This most often comes from the idea that the family is sacred and that one should not interfere with another person's family. It is also imperative to involve all team members in the decision to report an incident to the elder abuse hotline. This provides an opportunity to assess the situation from several different viewpoints and listen to other areas of concern. This, however, does not release the professional from his or her obligation to report suspected abuse because other team members may not agree. Professionals have an ethical, and in some situations, legal obligation to report elder abuse. If the client is in immediate danger, the police and the hotline should be called immediately. A caseworker is assigned to the case and sent out within 24 hours to complete a face-to-face interview. For most neglect and non-life threatening physical abuse reports the caseworker will usually interview the client within 72 hours of the report. For financial and psychological/emotional abuse the caseworker will interview the client within 7 days of the report.

In this case the team decided to report the abuse to the elder abuse hotline and inform them of its involvement with the family. The team would try to provide the family with services it felt could benefit all involved. The team decided that because they were going to be in contact with the family, to provide home health care services for 6-8 weeks that they would be able to impact and monitor the family's provision of services for Mrs. A.

Within 6 days of the elder abuse report, the caseworker was able to interview Mrs. A and requested permission to speak with the case manager of the home health care team, the nurse. The elder abuse caseworker found that the family was willing to work with them and did not refute the allegations made by the home health care team. The caseworker made suggestions similar to those of the home health care team and suggested that the client follow their recommendations. The caseworker also suggested to Mrs. A that she had the option to leave her daughter's home and that she could assist her in finding a nursing facility if she wished. Mrs. A declined moving to a nursing facility at that time.

Upon discharge from occupational therapy services, Mrs. A continued to utilize the home health aide 4 hours per day. Her daughter was pleased with her progress and was able to use the time that the home health aide was in the home to do things that she enjoyed; however, she continued to encourage her mother to discontinue her daily use of the home health aide. After 3-1/2 months, Mrs. A reduced the number of times the home health aide assisted her from 7 days per week to 5 days per week.

ELDER ABUSE HOTLINE INFORMATION

National Center on Elder Abuse
1225-I St., NW
Washington, DC 20005
Phone: 1-202-898-2586
Website: *http://www.gwjapan.com/NCEA*

U.S. Administration of Aging
Elder Care Locator number 1-800-677-1116
Contains information about state and local agencies, tribal organizations, and private organizations that serve the elderly in their communities or anywhere in the country.

REFERENCES

Ferguson, D., Beck, C. (1983). H.A.L.F.–A tool to assess elder abuse within the family. *Geriatric Nursing*, September/October, 301-314.
Fulmer, T.T., O'Malley, T.A. (1987). *Inadequate care of the elderly: A healthcare perspective on abuse and neglect*. New York: Springer Publishing.
Hamilton, G.P. (1989). Prevent elder abuse: Using a family systems approach. *Journal of Gerontological Nursing*, 15 (3), 21-26.
Hasselkus, B. (1991). Ethical dilemmas in family caregiving for the elderly: Implications for occupational therapy. *American Journal of Occupational Therapy*, 45, 206-212.

Haviland, S., O'Brien, J. (1989). Physical abuse and neglect of the elderly: Assessment and intervention. *Orthopaedic Nurse,* 8(4), 11-19.

Johnson, T. (1991). Elder mistreatment: Deciding who is at risk. Westport, CT: Greenwood Press.

King, M., Ryan, J. (1989). Abused women: Dispelling myths and encouraging intervention. *Nurse Practitioner,* 14(5), 47-58.

Kosberg, J.I. (1988). Preventing elder abuse: Identification of high risk factors to placement decisions. *Gerontologist,* 28, 43-50.

Larue, G.A. (1992). *Geroethics.* Buffalo, NY: Prometheus Books.

Moss, V., Taylor, W. (1991). Domestic violence: Identification, assessment, intervention. *AORN Journal,* 53(5), 1158-1164.

National Center on Elder Abuse at the American Public Human Services Association (NEAIS) (1998). The National Elder Abuse Incidence Study; Final Report, September 1998. *www.aoa.dhhs.gov/abuse/report/default.html.*

Pillemer, K., Finkelhor, D. (1988). The prevalence of elder abuse: A random sample survey. *Gerontologist,* 28, 51-57.

U.S. Congress, House select committee on aging (1990). *Elder abuse: A decade of shame and inaction.* Washington, DC: US Government Printing Office.

Index

ABA. *See* American Bar Association (ABA)
Abandonment
 defined, 12
 of the elderly, 144
Ability, defined, 39
Abuse
 alcohol, in identifying abuse, 19
 child. *See* Child abuse
 defining of, problems associated with, 144-145,145t-146t
 domestic. *See* Domestic abuse
 drug, in identifying abuse, 19
 economic, defined, 11
 elder. *See* Elder abuse
 emotional, defined, 10,12
 financial, of the elderly, 143
 history of, in identifying abuse, 19
 identification of, by occupational therapist, 15-17,19
 of people with disabilities, 8-9
 physical
  defined, 10,11
  of the elderly, 142-143
 psychological, of the elderly, 143
 sexual
  defined, 10-11,12-13
  of the elderly, 143
 spousal, knowledge and attitudes of occupational therapists regarding, 35-52. *See also* Wife abuse, knowledge and attitudes of occupational therapists regarding
 victims of, identification of, 13-17
 of wife. *See* Wife abuse
 of women, disclosure of, reluctance in, 14

Abuser(s), risk factors for becoming, 26-28
Academic Fieldwork Coordinator (AFC), 86
ACIS. *See* Assessment of Communication and Interaction Skills (ACIS)
Activity File, 87,89t
Adams, R., 15,35
Adolescent(s), domestic violence effects on, 20
Adult Protective Services, 29
AFC. *See* Academic Fieldwork Coordinator (AFC)
Alcohol abuse, in identifying abuse, 19
Allied Health Professions Project, 92
AMA. *See* American Medical Association (AMA)
American Academy of Family Physicians, 49
American Bar Association (ABA), 28
American Journal of Occupational Therapy, 16
American Medical Association (AMA), 36,49
American Occupational Therapy Association (AOTA), 40,41,48-49
American Physical Therapy Association (APTA), 48,49
AMPS. *See* Assessment of Motor and Process Skills (AMPS)
Analysis of variance (ANOVA), 44
ANOVA. *See* Analysis of variance (ANOVA)
Antisocial personality disorder, in identifying abuse, 19
Anxiety symptoms, in identifying abuse, 19
AOTA. *See* American Occupational Therapy Association (AOTA)

For Product Safety Concerns and Information please contact our
EU representative GPSR@taylorandfrancis.com Taylor & Francis
Verlag GmbH, Kaufingerstraße 24, 80331 München, Germany